CRITICAL ACCLAIM FOR THE WORKS OF JAMES RADA JR.

Canawlers

"Come 'canawling' with the Fitzgeralds and experience the joys and dangers of life on the C&O Canal. You'll almost hear the horn blowing as they approach another lock."

The Potomac Review

"A powerful, thoughtful and fascinating historical novel, *Canawlers* documents author James Rada, Jr. as a writer of considerable and deftly expressed storytelling talent."

Midwest Book Review

"James Rada, of Cumberland, has written a historical novel for high-schoolers and adults, which relates the adventures, hardships and ultimate tragedy of a family of boaters on the C&O Canal. ... The tale moves quickly and should hold the attention of readers looking for an imaginative adventure set on the canal at a critical time in history."

Along the Towpath

The Rain Man

"*The Rain Man* starts out with a bang and engages the reader with its fast-moving plot."
Beyond 50

"*The Rain Man* is a mystery thriller that races from the first raindrops that began the flooding to its dangerous climax in Wills Creek as it became a raging torrent."
Cumberland Times-News

Between Rail and River

"The book is an enjoyable, clean family read, with characters young and old for a broad-based appeal to both teens and adults. *Between Rail and River* also provides a unique, regional appeal, as it teaches about a particular group of people, ordinary working 'canawlers' in a story that goes beyond the usual coverage of life during the Civil War."
Historical Fiction Review

"*Between Rail and River* arrived yesterday – I finished it today. I couldn't put it down. Great job! … I enjoyed it thoroughly and I'm looking forward to the next installment."
Gary Petrichick
Author of *Pocket Guide to the Civil War on the Chesapeake and Ohio Canal*

Battlefield Angels

The Daughters of Charity Work as Civil War Nurses

by
James Rada, Jr.

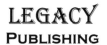

LEGACY
PUBLISHING

A division of AIM Publishing Group

BATTLEFIELD ANGELS:
THE DAUGHTERS OF CHARITY WORK AS CIVIL WAR NURSES

Published by Legacy Publishing, a division of AIM Publishing Group.
Gettysburg, Pennsylvania.
Copyright © 2011 by James Rada, Jr.
All rights reserved.
Printed in the United States of America.
First printing: August 2011.

ISBN 0-978-0-9714599-5-3

Cover design by James Rada, Jr. and Stephanie E. J. Long

Library of Congress Control Number: 2011917673

LEGACY
PUBLISHING

315 Oak Lane • Gettysburg, Pennsylvania 17325

Table of Contents

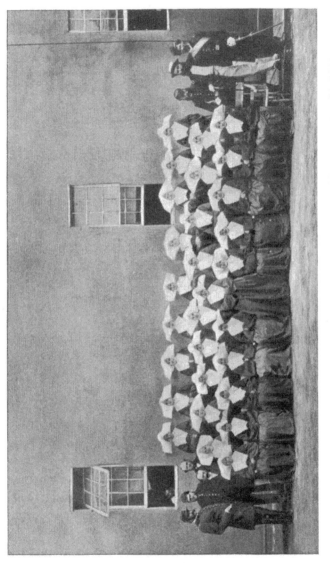

Daughters of Charity at Satterlee Military Hospital in Philadelphia during the Civil War. Courtesy of the Philadelphia Archdiocesan Historical Research Center.

Author's Introduction

"The country had only 600 trained nurses at the start of the Civil War. All were Catholic nuns. This is one of the best-kept secrets in our nation's history."

Father William Barnaby Faherty

As deadly as the Civil War was (620,000 dead and 282,000 wounded), it would have been much worse without the selfless help of Catholic sisters. These angels of the battlefield were so crucial to the survival of so many soldiers during the Civil War that I was surprised to find that more hadn't been written about them. As with most tales of war, the battles, charges, and heroics in the face of certain death make just about anything else pale in comparison.

Yet the battles to save lives are just as heroic, if not more noble, than the effort to take life and the Catholic sisters during the war were the heroines of these battles. With their wide, white cornettes looking almost like wings, the Daughters of Charity resembled angels gliding across the battlefield from man to man bringing comfort and relief. The sight of those wing-like cornettes told soldiers that relief was on the way; someone who cared for them was coming to help.

By focusing primarily on the American Daughters of Charity in this book, it is not my intention to slight the memory of the other two dozen or so orders of sisters who served during the war. I did it because the story of the Daughters of Charity tends to get lost amid the general story of Catholic sisters providing battlefield service as many times all Catholic sisters are grouped under "Sisters of Charity" or "Sisters of Mercy."

However, the different orders each had a different perspective on the war. The Daughters of Charity not only ran hospitals, served on troop transports, and provided care in battlefield hospitals, but they also cared for the sick and injured on both sides of the war and had their own Central House taken over by armies from both sides of the war.

While the soldiers came to respect the sisters because of the quality care they provided, the sisters measured their success by the number of baptisms that occurred among the soldiers. The Daughters of Charity were the most-experienced nurses in the country at the time of the Civil War, but the artillery shells fired from cannons could do even more damage than the sisters could help heal. If they engaged in battle with Satan for a soldier's soul, even if their earthly skills failed to heal a soldier's wounds, the sisters could still have the satisfaction of knowing that they had saved the soldiers' souls.

Most of the first-person accounts left by the Daughters of Charity reflect this attitude. I've chosen to look more at sisters' nursing talents and place their stories within the context of the war.

Though the Daughters of Charity trace their roots in North America as the Sisters of Charity of St. Joseph's in 1809, once the Emmitsburg-based community became affiliated itself with the Daughters of Charity in France in 1850, they took on that name. This is part of the reason for some of the confusion over where the Daughters of Charity served during the war. Even the sisters many times referred to themselves as Sisters of Charity rather than Daughters of Charity.

Living in Gettysburg, Pennsylvania, like I do, you can't avoid the Civil War. Gettysburg is frozen in that time period. You walk along streets and see re-enactors in costume marching along in front of you, shopping in stores and camping in fields. It seems that most of the land around the town has been designated part of the National Park Service's historic battlefield. When I first moved to the town, I knew something about the Battle of Gettysburg, but once I had lived there for a time, I began wondering what happened after the cannons fell silent and the armies marched away after three days of fighting and killing. With the casualties so high, who took care of the tens of thousands of dead and wounded? The battle may have lasted three days, but the recovery from the mammoth clash took much, much longer.

This is when I first heard about the Catholic sisters who helped care for the wounded, both in the emergency hospitals in and around Gettysburg and on the battlefield.

When I took a job a short distance south just over the Maryland border in Emmitsburg, Maryland, I began having contact with the Daughters of Charity who still have a strong presence in the town.

I slowly heard more stories and became fascinated by the extent of the work the sisters performed during the war. So good was their reputation, the Union and Confederate governments both requested their services.

Amazingly, the sisters had such a high level of trust among the government officials that they were allowed in the early part of the war to move back and forth across the border between the two warring countries. Nor did they betray that trust as they served officers and soldiers, Union and Confederate, with the same level of care.

This was all done in not only an environment of war but among a general social distaste against Catholics. However, as the Bible notes of charity, it "never faileth." In this way, the Daughters of Charity lived up to their name and broke down religious barriers even as the war that raged about them set brother against brother.

This is the story of their heavenly work and the fruits it bore.

James Rada, Jr.
June 1, 2011

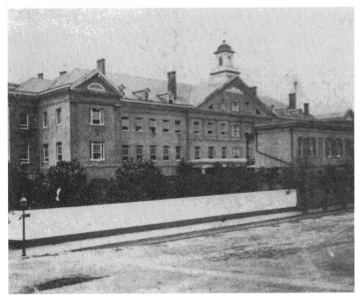

Charity Hospital in New Orleans. Louisiana paid the Daughters of Charity to staff and administer it. Courtesy of the Louisiana State Museum. (above) White House Landing eventually became the location for Arlington National Cemetery. The Daughters of Charity stayed here while they nursed the wounded soldiers. Courtesy of the Library of Congress. (below)

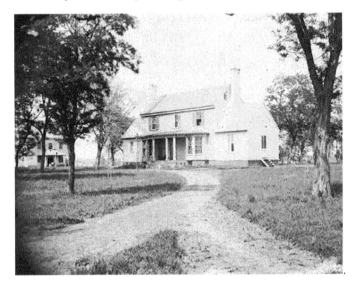

8

CHAPTER 1
Treason or Charity
.

*"On all of God's green and beautiful earth,
there are no purer, no nobler, no more kind-
hearted and self-sacrificing women than those
who wear the somber garb of the Catholic Sisters...Their only recompense, the sweet, soul-
soothing consciousness that they were doing
their duty; their only hope of reward, that peace
and eternal happiness which awaited them beyond the star-emblazoned battlements above."*

*Capt. Jack Crawford
Civil War Soldier and Poet*

Sister Regina Smith looked at the four men in front of her, letting the silence following their request become awkward. Not that she wanted to create that feeling. She was merely unsure how to respond. Best to say nothing than something that could cause an international incident...literally.

These men had ridden in their carriages from city hall on a spring afternoon on March 27, 1861, to meet with Sister Regina in her role as the administrator of Charity Hospital in New Orleans. Who they were has been lost to history, but they represented the governments of both New Orleans and the new Confederate nation[1] that had formed only the prior month within a couple of weeks of the inauguration of Abraham Lincoln as President of the United States.

One of the men would have undoubtedly been New Orleans Mayor John T. Monroe, a transplanted Virginian, who had been

James Rada, Jr.

elected in 1860. He would have been at the meeting representing the city's and state's interests since the State of Louisiana owned Charity Hospital.

Another one of Sister Regina's callers may have been Brigadier General Braxton Bragg, who had been promoted to his rank in the Confederate Army only a few weeks earlier. He commanded the Confederate forces around New Orleans and is known to have made the same request of the Daughters of Charity at this time,[2] but whether it was by letter, courier or in person is unknown.

The other two men may have been members of the Charity Hospital Board of Administrators. Since the Daughters of Charity did not own the hospital but only ran it for the State of Louisiana,[3] they reported to the board of directors.

Louisiana had seceded from the United States on January 26, 1861. It was the sixth state to do so, and since that time, Texas had also seceded. Now, this new confederation not only needed to find a way to work together when each believed that state took precedence over country, but they needed to re-establish the framework they had lost when they seceded, such as a military medical system to care for sick and wounded soldiers.

The Provisional Congress of the Confederate States of America had established its military structure on February 26, 1861. It had included a Medical Department, which at the time only had a surgeon general, four surgeons and six assistant surgeons to care for the thousands of soldiers in the regular army at the time.[4]

Help was needed, and since it would not be immediately forthcoming from the Confederate government, other avenues were being sought. These men—these representatives—had come with a single request, one which the Daughters of Charity seemed unable to deny whenever it was made: *Please, help us.*

They wanted the Daughters of Charity to help care for Confederates soldiers who were sick just as they cared for any person, rich or poor, young or old, white or black who came to Charity Hospital. Usually, this would have been an easy request for Sister Regina to answer. The mission of the Daughters of Charity was to perform "Works of piety, charity and usefulness and especially for the care of the sick, the succor of the aged and infirm and necessitous persons, and the education of young females."[5]

This request was different, though, because the soldiers were Confederate. Sister Regina was now technically serving in a foreign mission for the American Daughters of Charity who were based in Emmitsburg, Maryland. To act positively on the request could be construed as taking a side in the growing tensions between the Union and Confederate governments. That could create problems for the Central House, which was located in the Union. To not act, though, meant men could die. Men whose bodies...and souls...the Daughters of Charity could yet save.

Decision once again lay heavy upon Sister Regina's shoulders. It was a weight that had broken her health and led to her removal as the Mother Superior of the Daughters of Charity in 1859. She had served well and faithfully, but watching over hundreds of women spread across the country...drained a person. One biographer wrote, "...she had never been robust, and the responsibility she had borne during these years past, had exhausted her strength so that Superiors felt obliged to relieve her of the cross not too heavy for her enfeebled condition."[6]

Sister Regina Smith was fifty-four years old in 1861, an old woman in the eyes of many. In her more than thirty-eight years as a Sister and then Daughter of Charity, she and Death had become familiar acquaintances but never friends. No never friends. Even before she had become Mother Superior to the Daughters of Charity, she had seen sisters die...her real sister, friends and sisters in God in 1832. Each of their deaths had taken something from her, and she had not even been responsible for them. How much more it had pained her when she was Mother and had sent sisters away to serve only to have them die!

Yet, those sisters had served faithfully to the end, knowing they were where their God wanted them to be and if they gave their lives in His service, so much the sooner they would join him. Could Sister Regina do any less now that she was merely a sister? Mother Ann Simeon Norris, Sister Regina's replacement, had sent her to New Orleans because this was where she needed to be now. Sister Regina had been born in Louisiana. She had served for years here including facilitating the assumption of responsibility for Charity Hospital for the Daughters of Charity.

If time had allowed, Sister Regina would have notified Mother Ann Simeon at the Central House in Emmitsburg, but to wait for a decision could take days that the sick soldiers might not have. Was it not the duty of a sister to strive to fulfill the mission of the Daughters of Charity wherever the opportunity existed?

To this, there was but one answer, and it was the same answer she gave the men who were sitting her office. *Yes.* Yes, the Daughters of Charity would nurse their soldiers. Four sisters were sent to care for wounded and sick soldiers in Pensacola and Warrington, Florida.[7] Sister Regina also later sent four sisters from Charity Hospital to care for wounded Confederate soldiers and those suffering from "malignant fevers" at Camp Moore near Kentwood, Louisiana, about eighty-six miles from New Orleans.[8]

And with this action, the Daughters of Charity took a first tentative step that would eventually have hundreds of sisters caring for tens of thousands of soldiers who became casualties of the Civil War.

Jane Columba Loretto Smith had thought that the worst day in her life was the day her parents died. It was a private pain she carried in her heart, releasing it only when she lit a candle for each of her parents and prayed for them. Each time she remembered her parents, she found the memories a little less painful.

Jane grew up in Grand Coteau, Louisiana, a small village that was not much more than a stagecoach stopover. It also had a few other businesses; the inn where the stage stopped, a post office, a blacksmith shop, millinery, a cobbler and two bakeries. Jane turned fifteen years old in 1821. That was also the year she lost her parents.

When her parents had died, most likely taken by one of the contagious diseases that periodically swept through the area, caring for Jane and her younger sister, Mary Ann, had fallen to their uncle, Raphael Smith. Being a pious man, he turned the care of his nieces over to the Sisters of Charity in Emmitsburg and allowed the proceeds from his brother's estate to pay for their education at the school.[9]

It was not an unusual decision for him to make. His own sister had already taken the vows of a Sister of Charity and was serving at St. Joseph's Academy.[10] He would also send his own daughter to St. Joseph's in 1830.[11]

The school had opened in 1809 as a free school, but financial problems required the Sisters of Charity to begin accepting paying students. The school had quickly outgrown its original building and had moved into St. Joseph's House, a substantial log house that was covered in clapboards and painted white.[12] Young women learned reading, spelling, grammar, and mathematics in their core classes and then they could choose elective courses that included needlework, music, and languages.[13]

By the time the Smith sisters arrived in Emmitsburg, St. Joseph's House was filled to bursting with boarding students, sisters and day students. The Sisters of Charity were working through a transition period. Mother Elizabeth Ann Seton, who had founded the order in 1809, died on January 4, 1821, around nine months before the Smith sisters arrived.

Mother Rose White had been chosen to serve as the new Mother Superior for the Sisters of Charity at the end of January and returned from the mission field to assume her new duties in Emmitsburg in March. Sister Margaret George was called as the directress of St. Joseph's Academy.[14]

Jane thrived under the tutelage of the sisters, and with them as her role models, she sought admittance to the Sisters of Charity. The sisters received her as a candidate on July 12, 1823, when she was not yet seventeen years old. Once she had completed a three-month probation, Jane took on the name Regina and began wearing a novice's habit.[15]

Two years later, Sister Regina's actual sister, Mary Ann, was admitted to the Sisters of Charity as a novice. However, within days of this good news, Mary Ann was caught in a severe storm far from the academy with children whom she had decided to take on a long, long walk. Rushing to get back to the academy, she had carried one of the smaller children the entire distance. The next day, Mary Ann was unable to rise from her bed, and she was cold to the touch. The sisters administered to her, but the worst was feared, and Father Gabriel Brute´ arrived from nearby Mount St. Mary's College to give the young sister Last Rites.

Sister Regina suffered another significant loss when her sister died on July 19, 1825, with Sister Regina sitting at her bedside.[16]

Father Brute´ wrote, "This young girl of eighteen, but three days ago in perfect health, now dying far from home – her own dear sister at her side. But, O my God! What joy in seeing a good, holy soul preparing with such pious simplicity and calm obedience to meet her Lord, to enter another world and begin her eternity."[17]

Sister Regina took her first vows as a Sister of Charity the following year on March 15.

In 1829, Bishop Joseph Rosati asked for help from the Sisters of Charity in New Orleans. He was serving as both the bishop of Saint Louis, Missouri, and the administrator of the Diocese of New Orleans at the time. His time and attention were stretched thin, and the sisters had previously helped him in St. Louis, so he valued their aid.

Sister Regina and Sister Magdallen Councell Emmitsburg on December 29, traveled to Baltimore and from there, sailed to New Orleans arriving on January 30, 1830, but not without some adventure on their journey.

Their vessel was pursued by pirates during seven hours;

all on board were in consternation except those who relied on their omnipotent, heavenly Protector. On another occasion they had the sorrow to meet a small vessel in frightful distress, many of the passengers being very ill; but the heart of good Sister Regina suggested means of comforting and relieving them.[18]

The two sisters stayed with the Ursuline nuns who had a convent in the city. The sisters taught young, black girls at a school that had been privately established there. Their success there led to more requests to teach at other schools and more sisters in the New Orleans.

It also resulted in another important assignment for Sister Regina. In May 1833, the Charity Hospital Board of Directors, impressed by the work of the Sisters of Charity, wrote to the Central House:

> Respected Sisters, The high reputation for humanity and devotion to the indigent which the ladies of the institute over which you reside have acquired has been represented to the board of administrators of the Charity Hospital of this city and has made it advisable to them to obtain sisters to manage the interior economy of the institution…. It is to supersede and take under your immediate management the household concern of the hospital that we are desirous to employ the sisters. The number we require will be about 10 and the remuneration they will receive will be, if satisfactory to them, regulated by the same terms as those who are engaged in the F. Markham Asylum of this city.[19]

Charity Hospital had been founded in 1736 using funds bequeathed in the will of French sailor and shipbuilder Jen Louis who died in New Orleans in 1735. The hospital's primary mission was to serve the poor, which coincided with the mission of

15

the Sisters of Charity. As the hospital grew, it relocated and expanded into larger facilities. The fifth hospital building was built in 1832 in the Faubourg St. Marie, shortly before the board of administrators decided that they needed better management for the hospital.

The actual remuneration the board of directors offered the Sisters of Charity was $150 a year, and the sisters could live in the hospital. The hospital also owned sixteen slaves who would perform the menial work leaving the sisters free to care for the sick.[20]

Sister Regina and nine other sisters assumed control of Charity Hospital on January 6, 1834. At the time, 180 patients were in the hospital, and many of them were considered insane.[21] The hospital itself was three stories tall with ten halls, five surgical wards, and accommodations for 540 patients.[22]

Within a few months, yellow fever began striking down residents. Yellow fever is a disease transmitted by mosquitoes, which were plentiful in bayous of Louisiana. However, the fact that mosquitos were the carrier would not be suspected until 1881, and then it would still be more than another decade before it was proven.[23] Besides fever, other symptoms included nausea and pain. In later stages, the liver can be damaged, which leads to jaundice and the reason for "yellow" in the name. People feared yellow fever and with good reason. It was a deadly disease at the time with a high mortality rate. A history of the city noted, "New Orleans streets were deserted; stores were closed; people remaining in the city, huddled in their houses, making pitiful attempts to fight off the disease. It was a city of the dead."[24]

Sister Regina and the sisters under her administration fought against the disease, caring for the sick and seeing little in the way of results. The number of cases at the hospital spiked so sharply that Sister Regina wrote to the Central House asking for ten more sisters to assist her at Charity Hospital. They were sent, but by the time they arrived in November 1834, five of the original ten sisters had died from yellow fever. Two of the replacement group also died within the next six months.[25]

Sister Regina continued working at Charity Hospital until 1854 and "Under Sister Regina's leadership, the sisters strove to improve their nursing skills, with the older and more experienced on the wards teaching their younger and newer partners all that they had learned."[26]

Following her assignment in New Orleans, she traveled to France where she stayed at the Mother House of the Daughters of Charity there, with whom the Sisters of Charity had affiliated themselves in 1850. During her time there, she came to personally know the superiors of the Daughters of Charity as they came to know her. When Sister Regina returned to the United States in 1855, she was appointed Visitatrix of the American Daughters of Charity and took the title Mother.

In his letter appointing her, Superior General Jean-Baptiste Étienne wrote in part, "Having had the opportunity of seeing her, and of appreciating the excellent qualities of her mind, I felt convinced that God called her to conduct your Province in the path of perfection which has opened before you, and in the accomplishment of the destiny reserved for you."[27]

As she assumed the leadership role for the Daughters of Charity, the Central House was receiving more and more calls for help either as teachers or nurses across the country. Mother Regina responded with help as best she could, and under her guidance, the Daughters of Charity began opening hospitals and schools across the country.

As Mother Regina sent the sisters out to serve, she must have realized that some might not ever return to the Central House, which was the case. All of these deaths weighed heavily on Mother Regina to the point that her health began to fail. "But the health of dear Mother Regina was much impaired; she had never been robust, and the responsibility she had borne during these years past, had exhausted her strength, so that Superiors felt obliged to relieve her of the cross now too heavy for her enfeebled condition."[28]

James Rada, Jr.

Though Mother, now Sister Regina was no longer the leader of the Daughters of Charity, she still had skills, knowledge, and experience that made her invaluable for what the sisters were about to face.

She was happy when she was called once again to serve as the administrator for Charity Hospital, but it was a decision made not so much to please Sister Regina as to place her where she would be able to provide the most service.

This she proved when she became the first contact that the Daughters of Charity had with the opposing governments of the United States of America and the Confederate States of America on March 27, 1861.

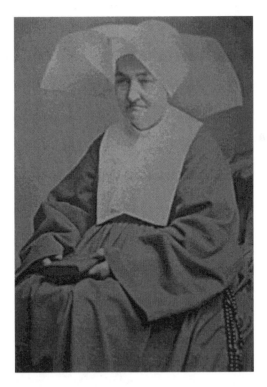

Sister Mary Louise Caulfield. Photo courtesy of the Daughters of Charity.

CHAPTER 2
A House Divided

*"The Catholic Sisters were the most efficient ...
veritable Angels of Mercy."*

Lucius Chittenden
U.S. Register of the Treasury

With the inauguration of Jefferson Davis as the president of the Confederate States of American on February 18, 1861, the United States had become two separate countries. During his inaugural address, he repeatedly spoke that the Confederate States existed because the United States had failed to recognize the right of the states and individuals to govern themselves as outlined in the U.S. Constitution. He spoke of living in peace with the North and establishing trade between the sibling countries, but he also said the Confederate States would defend the rights which the Southern States had sought to preserve through secession.

Our present position has been achieved in a manner unprecedented in the history of nations. It illustrates the American idea that government rests upon the consent of the governed, and that it is the right of the people to alter or abolish a government whenever it becomes destructive of the ends for which it was established. The declared purposes of the compact of Union from which we have withdrawn were to establish justice, insure domestic tranquility, to provide for the common defense, to promote the general welfare, and to secure the blessings

19

of liberty for ourselves and our posterity; and when in the judgment of the sovereign States now comprising this Confederacy it had been perverted from the purposes for which it was ordained, and had ceased to answer the ends for which it was established, an appeal to the ballot box declared that so far as they were concerned the government created by that compact should cease to exist. In this they merely asserted a right which the Declaration of Independence of 1776 defined to be inalienable.[43]

Two weeks later, Abraham Lincoln was inaugurated as President of the much-diminished United States. So tense and uncertain the times were that Lincoln, all the while guarded by General Winfield Scott's soldiers, took a secret route to Washington for his inauguration. He took the oath of office on the east portico of the Capitol Building, which was covered in scaffolding because the wood-and-copper dome was being replaced by a cast iron one.

The new President sought to assure Southern citizens that he would not interfere with slavery where it already existed, but he did not recognize the legitimacy of the Confederate States. Lincoln said in his inaugural address:

But if destruction of the Union by one or by a part only of the States be lawfully possible, the Union is less perfect than before the Constitution, having lost the vital element of perpetuity.

It follows from these views that no State upon its own mere motion can lawfully get out of the Union; that resolves and ordinances to that effect are legally void, and that acts of violence within any State or States against the authority of the United States are insurrectionary or revolutionary, according to circumstances.

I therefore consider that in view of the Constitution

and the laws the Union is unbroken, and to the extent of my ability, I shall take care, as the Constitution itself expressly enjoins upon me, that the laws of the Union be faithfully executed in all the States. Doing this I deem to be only a simple duty on my part, and I shall perform it so far as practicable unless my rightful masters, the American people, shall withhold the requisite means or in some authoritative manner direct the contrary. I trust this will not be regarded as a menace, but only as the declared purpose of the Union that it will constitutionally defend and maintain itself.[44]

Lincoln said he believed that all the laws of the land should be enforced in all the states. If that meant returning a runaway slave to his or her owner, so be it. If it meant collecting a tariff in a state claiming secession, so be it.

The uneasy and tenuous peace between the Union and the Confederacy lasted less than three months and about two weeks after the Confederate States of America had asked for the help of the Daughters of Charity.

On April 12, 1861, Brigadier General P. G. T. Beauregard of the Confederate Army bombarded Fort Sumter in Charleston Harbor in South Carolina for more than thirty hours and forced the surrender of the federal fort on April 13. Thus, began the Civil War.

Three days later, President Lincoln asked for 75,000 volunteers to uphold the United States of America.

Responding to Lincoln's request for volunteers, Virginia seceded on April 17, Arkansas on May 6, Tennessee on May 7, and North Carolina on May 20. Kentucky adopted a resolution of neutrality on May 20. One day later, Richmond, Virginia, became the capital of the Confederacy. In June, the people of western Virginia convened in Wheeling, Virginia, and set up a Unionist government.

* * *

21

James Rada, Jr.

As the United States broke apart, Daughters of Charity from Emmitsburg found themselves serving God in two countries. In the United States, they were divided among New York, Massachusetts, Pennsylvania, Wisconsin, Michigan, Illinois, Maryland, and California. In the Confederate States, they served in Louisiana, Mississippi, Alabama, Missouri, and Virginia.

Though the Sisters and Daughters of Charity had been in existence for fifty-two years in 1861, their mother organization had been around since 1617 when Saint Vincent de Paul formed the first lay confraternity of charity for women which later developed into the Ladies of Charity. Not long after their founding, Saint Vincent told the sisters, "Men go to war to kill one another, and you, sisters, you go to repair the harm they had have done... Men kill the body and very often the soul, and you go to restore life, or at least by your care to assist in preserving it."[45]

The Daughters of Charity in Europe had lived up to this mission during the Crimean War when England, France, and Sardinia helped Turkey defend itself against Russia. The Daughters of Charity worked as nurses with the French soldiers, easing their pains and caring for the soldiers until they were healthy again.

During the war, the British quickly became dismayed at the conditions sick and wounded British soldiers were forced to endure. War correspondent Thomas Chenery had brought the plight of the British troops to light in his battle reports and pointed out the excellent care the French received. He wrote in his newspaper report, "Why have we no Sisters of Charity?"[46] It was a rallying call for better battlefield nursing care.

Yet, even proper nursing care in hospitals at the time was still in its infancy. It was believed by many that nursing was not a suitable profession for women, so nursing in public hospitals was often done by other residents of the hospital or the poor. No formal training program existed, and most nurses either learned their skills by providing care to family members or assisting a doctor to whom they were related.

The Sisters of Charity in America entered into health care

when they took over the management of nursing services of the Baltimore Infirmary in 1823, and five years later, they opened the first Catholic hospital west of the Mississippi River. The Sisters of Charity continued to grow. In 1850, when they affiliated themselves with the Mother House of the Daughters of Charity in Paris, they adopted the blue-gray dress, white collar and white cornette that would eventually distinguish them as unique. They also took the name of their mother organization becoming Daughters, rather than Sisters, of Charity.

This French affiliation created its own civil war within the order of sisters. Sister Margaret Cecilia George oversaw a branch of the Sisters of Charity in Cincinnati, Ohio. She was the last remaining of the original eighteen Sisters of Charity who were with Mother Elizabeth Ann Seton when they were professed by Baltimore Archbishop John Carroll in 1813 and felt that the affiliation was an abandonment of what Mother Seton had established. Five sisters whom she oversaw also felt this way.[47]

Archbishop of Cincinnati John Baptist Purcell took up the cause with his fellow clergymen and on February 25, 1852, told the Sisters of Charity of Cincinnati that they could continue to follow their traditional ways. They could establish a new Mother House in Cincinnati and that he would serve as their spiritual leader.[48]

> They knew well what was being taken from them; they did not forget that the strength of their young lives had gone into the building up of all the institutions then doing the work planned by their founders; they knew the old familiar garb of Mother Seton was to be banished from the old familiar places and that unless God's blessing would fall upon the colonies in New York and Cincinnati and multiply the families, the pioneer community of the United States would be an event of the past.[49]

A seventh sister from New Orleans and novices soon joined

them. Sister Margaret became Mother Margaret, the first mother-superior of the Sisters of Charity of Cincinnati on February 7, 1853.[50]

As the Civil War approached, the Daughters of Charity continued their work among the sick whoever they might be. They gained experience working with victims of violence, accidents, and cholera in Baltimore, Philadelphia and Boston during outbreaks in 1832-1833 and 1850.

> The zeal with which these important duties were performed, entitles those pious ladies to the highest praise from all humane persons, and has deeply impressed upon the members of this Board's feelings of high respect, and obtained their most sincere thanks.[51]

The Daughters of Charity also cared for patients with yellow fever in the South during a 1855 outbreak. These varied experiences in dangerous surroundings became the training ground for what they would face in the war. "What the prevailing opinion overlooked, however, was that sisters brought something to the battlefields that was rare: more nursing experience than the armies have," noted one modern historian who wrote of Sister-nurses.[52]

As the expectation of a war between the Union and Confederacy grew, it became apparent that the Daughters of Charity and some of the other Catholic sisterhoods were the only sources for trained nurses.[53]

Professional nurses were virtually unheard of at the time. It was considered unladylike for women to care for men the way nurses needed to. Bathing men who weren't their husbands was something only women of ill repute would do. Male doctors worried that women would faint at the sight of the blood and gore.[54] Even in the army where care was needed more frequently, nursing care was generally done by other patients who were further along in their recovery.[55]

However, despite the reticence people had about the Catholic religion at the time, they showed little of that hesitation in accepting the care that the Daughters of Charity and other Catholic sisters offered. Mary Livermore, who worked with a sanitary commission during the war, wrote years later:

> I am neither a Catholic, nor an advocate of the monastic institutions of that church. Similar organizations established on the basis of the Protestant religion, and in harmony with republican principles, might be made very helpful to modern society, and would furnish occupation and give position to large numbers of unmarried women, whose hearts go out to the work in charitable intent. But I can never forget my experience during the War of Rebellion. Never did I meet these Catholic sisters in hospitals, on transports, on hospital steamers, without observing their devotion, faithfulness, and unobtrusiveness. They gave themselves no airs of superiority or holiness, shirked no duty, sought no easy place, bred no mischiefs. Sick and wounded men watched for their entrance into the wards at morning, and looked a regretful farewell when they departed at night. They broke down in exhaustion from overwork, as did the Protestant nurses; like them, they succumbed to the fatal prison-fever, which our exchanged prisoners brought from the fearful pens of the South.[56]

Such was the country broken, and the Daughters of Charity would help heal it one body and one soul at a time.

James Rada, Jr.

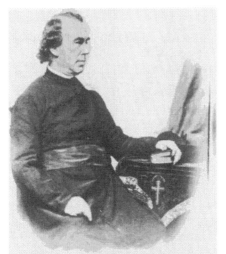

Father James Francis Burlando, director of the Daughters of Charity during the Civil War. (above) Mother Ann Simeon led the American Daughters of Charity during the Civil War. Courtesy of the Daughters of Charity (below).

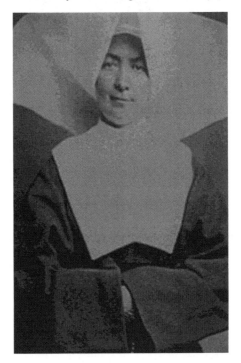

CHAPTER 3
Care as an Afterthought

"My most sincere and hearty thanks for the faith-
ful and efficient manner in which you have per-
formed your duties. Joining it [Satterlee Hospital]
at its foundation under an impulse of true Chris-
tian charity you have remained true and stedfast
[sic] to the end; suffering discomfort, working
early and late, never murmuring. You have won
my gratitude and the gratitude of every true sol-
dier, and have confirmed me in the profound es-
teem which I have always entertained for your
noble order. ... May the knowledge of the good
which you have done to the sick and wounded and
weary soldiers of our common country be to you a
satisfaction and reward."

Surgeon Isaac Hayes
Satterlee Hospital

While the Union and the Confederacy may have been ready to fight and kill each other, they weren't prepared to care for those who survived the battles wounded and maimed. The U.S. Army medical staff had only eighty-seven personnel. There had been the surgeon general, thirty surgeons, and eighty-three assistant surgeons, but twenty-four of them had resigned their positions to return to their homes in the Confederate States, and three others were discharged for disloyalty.

Further south, the Confederate Army absorbed state militias of the Confederate States, each of which had a surgeon and assistant surgeon among their members. So as far as the number of medical personnel went, the Confederate Army looked great compared to the Union Army. The problem was that most of the Confederate surgeons and assistant surgeons were not always fully trained, let alone doctors who had experience treating war wounds.

Daniel DeLeon had been a U.S. Army surgeon who joined the Confederacy immediately and had taken any medical supplies with him that he could when he left his position with the U.S. Army. He saw nothing wrong with the action because in his view the Confederacy owned a portion of all federal property. He was merely taking the portion that belonged to the Confederate States and returning the supplies to their rightful owners.

DeLeon was from South Carolina, but he had received his medical training in Pennsylvania. He was appointed as the Confederate States' Acting Surgeon General on May 6, 1861. This was the beginning of the Confederate Medical Department. Yet it was a small start with only twenty-nine doctors and surgeons by the time the war officially broke out. The Confederate Congress had only allocated $350,000 for medical services. DeLeon used most of the money to acquire buildings in Richmond that could be used as hospitals.

Within two weeks of the beginning of the Civil War, 20,000-plus aid societies were established to help the soldiers and sailors who were protecting their country, be it Union or Confederate. Not all of the societies would continue for the full length of the war, but some would become very successful in their efforts.[1]

Recognizing the need to coordinate the efforts of the aid societies and manage the women volunteering to be nurses, U.S. Secretary of War Simon Cameron appointed Dorothea L. Dix, a Boston schoolteacher, as the superintendent of the U.S. Army nurses on April 23, 1861. Dix, who was a 60-year-old spinster, had earned a national reputation for two years of work in improving the conditions of the mentally ill. Cameron announced her service by writing:

The free services of Miss D. L. Dix are accepted by the War Department and that she will give at all times all necessary and in organizing military hospitals for the cure of all sick and wounded soldiers, aiding the chief surgeon by supplying nurses and substantial means for the comfort and relief of the suffering; also that she is fully authorized to receive, control, and disburse special supplies bestowed by individuals or associations for the comfort of their friends or the citizen soldiers from all parts of the limited states; as also, under section of the Acting Surgeon-General, to draw from army stores.[2]

Dix took to the work immediately giving directions about supplies, equipment, and operations. She traveled between the military hospitals to see what supplies each hospital had on hand. If a hospital was found lacking, she would fill out the supplies from the stores she kept in a house she rented.[3]

She also took steps to weed out women whom she thought would harm the reputation of her nurses. No woman under thirty years old need apply to serve in the government hospitals. All nurses were required to be plain-looking women. Their dresses had to be brown or black with no bows, no curls in their hair, no jewelry, and no hoop skirts. But for these requirements, there may have been more women accepted as nurses. In fact, Mary Walker, a female Civil War doctor saw Dix turn away potential nurses, "telling them that they were too young and too good-looking and when they told her what their ages were she disputed their word and they left."[4] Nurse Jane Woolsey said, "Society just now presents the unprecedented spectacle of many women trying to make-believe that they are over thirty!"[5]

Though these requirements would seem to fit many of the Catholic sisters and nuns serving in the war, Dix also had a "no Catholics need apply" proviso.[6]

One thing that may explain this proviso, other than the socie-

James Rada, Jr.

tal prejudice against Catholics, is that Dix had seen the charitable hospitals run by the Daughters of Charity in Paris in 1855 and come away less than overawed. She applauded the government support of the hospitals, but noted they had "two radical universal defects, at least."[7] These were poor ventilation and the experimental treatment methods used by the interns. She also expressed some distaste for the Catholic personnel at the hospital, writing:

> In *all* these establishments, associated with other employees, are found Sisters of Charity, and nuns of various orders. Some of them are very self-denying, not many. They are never overtasked, except possibly in some period of serious epidemic. As for the priests, they should for the most part occupy places in houses of correctional discipline, and enlightening cultivation.[8]

While Dix was less-than-impressed with the care the Sisters of Charity had offered, not everyone was impressed with Dix's work either. Dr. Walker watched Dix tour a hospital once and wrote of Dix:

> When she saw a patient who was too ill to arrange the clothing on his cot if it became disarranged and a foot was exposed she turned her head the other way seeming not to see the condition while I was so disgusted with such sham modesty that I hastened to arrange the soldier's bed clothing if I had a chance to be near when no nurses were to do this duty. I was not able to understand and am not to the present day of what use any one can be who professes to work for a cause and then allows sham modesty to prevent them from doing little services that chance to come their way.[9]

Another reason for Dix's opposition to Catholic involvement

could have been her second goal, which was to bring all unregulated nursing activities throughout the country under her control.[10] However, in developing a nursing care system that met with her approval, Dix stepped on more than a few toes among officers, doctors, and medical directors. Since the Catholic sisters were not under the jurisdiction of Dix, it made them an attractive alternative to use as nurses among men who didn't want to have to deal with Dix's demanding nature.

While Dix didn't want Catholic sisters helping with nursing, doctors on both sides of the fighting did. The Daughters of Charity work running hospitals and helping the sick during outbreaks of cholera and yellow fever in the previous decade were well known. It was also known that the Daughters of Charity were trained as nurses and not simply well-intentioned women.

Dix and her nurses were seen as stubborn and demanding by many doctors. Dr. John H. Brinton was the physician in charge at the Mound City Hospital at Mound City, Illinois. He wrote of his experience with Dix's nurses:

On the arrival of certain trains they [the nurses] would stalk into the office of district commanders, and establish themselves solemnly against the walls, entrenched behind their bags and parcels. They defied all military law. There they were, and there they would stay, until some accommodation might be found for them.[11]

He noted that the nurses were usually sent to the adjutant general, who would, in turn, send the women to the physician in charge of the hospital, such as he was. Brinton wrote sarcastically, "They [the nurses] did not wish much, not they, simply a room, a bed, a looking glass, someone to get their meals and do little things for them, and they would nurse the sick boys of our gallant Union Army."[12]

Though it sounds as if he were against all women nurses, he wasn't. He only frowned on those who used up his hospital's

James Rada, Jr.

scarce resources without providing a greater return for the wounded and sick soldiers. He found the nurses to be complainers, backbiters and fault finders. However, Brinton was pleased when fifteen Catholic sisters arrived to help, and the Mother Superior told him that all they needed was single room for all the sisters.[13] Though Brinton doesn't say which Catholic sisterhood the women were from, he does note that the appeal for nurses was made to the Catholic authorities in South Bend, Indiana, so it is likely the sisters were Sisters of the Holy Cross in that city.

While Dix was still organizing her nurses, the Catholic sisters were already at work on the battlefields. Battlefield healthcare was as dangerous to a soldier's health as battle wounds. Around 60 percent of the casualties during the war came from infectious diseases like dysentery, typhus, malaria, smallpox, measles, and tuberculosis because medicine at the time knew little about caring for infections.[14] By the end of the war, they would serve as nurses, hospital administrators, cooks, laundresses, dieticians, and apothecaries.

What would become quickly apparent is that the sisters brought more than physical relief to those they treated. Their patients recognized this even if the non-Catholics the sisters worked with didn't understand it.

Abby Hopper Gibbons was a Quaker who served as a nurse during the war. She wrote of a soldier at Point Lookout who told her, "Sisters, but they never enter into conversation with a soldier, and are, in consequence, but little comfort to the sick, while they work their machinery very well. All the sick are on our side."[15]

Either this was an isolated case, or Hopper was expressing an anti-Catholic bias that she shared with much of the country at the time. The Daughters of Charity were women to whom sick and wounded soldiers could talk. Soldiers entrusted them with their hopes and fears. Louisa May Alcott, the author of *Little Women*, served as a nurse in Washington City during the war. She de-

32

scribed this effect, saying, "And now I knew that to him, as to so many, I was the poor substitute for mother, wife, or sister, and in his eyes no stranger, but a friend who hitherto had seemed neglectful."[16]

In the Missouri Military Hospital in St. Louis where the Daughters of Charity not only performed nursing duties but also administered the hospital, a sister on her nightly rounds came upon a soldier who was suffering from pain in his forehead and temples. He had caught a cold in the camp, and the inflammation spread to his eyes to the point where they had swollen until he could no longer see. The soldier said the pain was so intense that he thought he wouldn't live until morning. The sister asked the man to allow her to bind his head with a wide bandage.

"Oh, Sister, it is no use," the man told her, his voice straining with desperation. "The doctor has been bathing my forehead with spirits of ether and other liquids, and nothing will do me any good. I cannot live until morning; my head is splitting open. But you may do what you like."

The sister took a wide bandage, and unknown to the soldier saturated it in chloroform. She bound up the man's head and left him for the night once the chloroform had eased him into sleep.

The next morning she returned and asked him how his night had been.

"Oh, Sister, I have rested well; from the moment you put your hands on my forehead I experienced no pain,"[17] the grateful patient told her.

Wise surgeons recognized this respect towards the sisters and used it to help their patients. Where a patient might reject a doctor's ministrations, it was not so with the sisters. Once treated, if the patient recovered, the sister got the credit, which only added to the power of their reputations and their ability to help others.

During another incident at the St. Louis Military Hospital, the sisters were walking through the wards when a soldier raised himself up in bed and said, "Ah, sister, how glad I am to see you. Ah! If you were here to take care of us, that poor boy" – He pointed to the soldier in the next bed. – "would be well long ago."[18]

One of the sisters serving at the hospital wrote:

> Some of them looked upon the sisters as superior beings. They said they could not understand how persons could live in the world and not care for the world. One man expressed himself thus (and he was a non-Catholic) that the Daughters of Charity were like gold tried in the fire.[19]

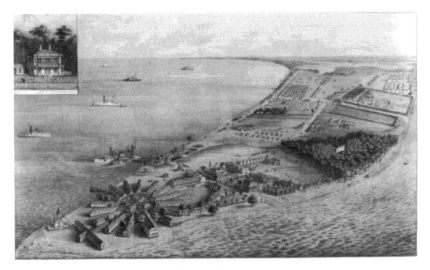

A bird's eye view of Point Lookout, Maryland. Hammond Hospital is the star-shaped set of buildings in the lower left. Courtesy of the Library of Congress.

CHAPTER 4
Guardian Angel of the Daughters of Charity

*"One of the things that impressed me was that
the Sisters made no distinction whatever between
the most polished gentlemen and the greatest
rapscallion in the lot; the measure of their
attention was solely the human suffering to be
relieved; and a miserable wretch in pain was a
person of more consequence to the Sisters than
the best of us when comparatively comfortable."*

Lieutenant Colonel Daniel Shipman Troy
60ᵗʰ Alabama Regiment

Mother Regina Smith still led the Daughters of Charity in the
years prior to war, but almost as if in anticipation of the future
stresses of the office, Father Francis Burlando, the director of the
Daughters of Charity, announced Sister Ann Simeon Norris as
the new Visitatrix of the Daughters of Charity on December 28,
1859.

"The majority of the Sisters had no intimation of the new appointment, although it would seem that the failing health of our
beloved Mother Regina Smith should have prepared them for the
change."[1]

Father James Francis Burlando entered the Daughters of
Charity Community Room at two o'clock on December 28. The
sisters who had gathered there fell silent and turned to face him.
With little fanfare, Father Burlando presented Mother Ann Simeon to the sisters. Though unsure of accepting the responsibility

35

"she offered no resistance but yielded herself a willing victim for the Community so dear to her heart."[2]

Mother Regina did not attend the announcement of her replacement. It was said that the new visitatrix looked slightly ill as she assumed the mantle of leadership among the sisters, but Father Burlando seemed quite happy with the change.[3]

Mother Ann Simeon had been born Louisa A. Norris on September 25, 1816, in Charles County, Maryland. She grew up in a prosperous life, "although not in affluent circumstances, they enjoyed all the comforts of an easy country life and had slaves to cultivate their farm which annually increased the income of the small family consisting of Louisa and two sons."[4]

Louisa's mother, Delia Tiers Norris, took great efforts to shape her only daughter's character. Once, when Louisa threw a temper tantrum, her mother corrected her.

"No one but you finds fault with me," Louisa said.

"My child, I correct you because I do not wish anyone else to see a fault in you," Mrs. Norris told her daughter.[5]

When Delia Norris died in 1834, Louisa left home for Washington to attend college. It was in Washington among similarly minded friends that Louisa decided to join the Sisters of Charity.

"Do you think I could be a sister?" Louisa asked her friends at one point.

They advised her to continue to improve herself and to wait until spring, and they would all join together. Louisa told her friends:

If they will take me as I am, I will go at once; you know, if I wait until spring, I shall have spent a portion of my funds, and perhaps I would not have sufficient to procure an outfit and meet necessary expenses. Oh, I cannot think of going to school now; but I will do all that depends on me to become a Sister of Charity. Should I be obliged to wait, I will in the meantime by my exertions, obtain the means necessary to secure admission when our Lord's time comes.[6]

However, Louisa's confessor also advised her to wait and so, she did not apply for the sisterhood until February 1835. She made her submission and waited anxiously for the answer, but it was not the one she had hoped for. Louisa's application was rejected because of her fragile health.

Louisa persisted, and the confessor priest took her case before Sister Martha Daddisman, the sister servant (or local superior) at Saint Vincent's Asylum, an orphanage and maternity hospital in Washington. The priest also advised Louisa to say the Thirty Days' Prayer for her particular intention.

The young girl did so and also worked to take better care of herself. At the end of that time, her health was much better, and the letter arrived accepting her application to the Sisters of Charity.

In his letter to Mother Rose White at St. Joseph's announcing the group of young postulants, Father William Mathews of Saint Patrick's Church in Washington wrote:

And lastly Louisa A. Norris in whom you will find the simplicity of the dove, the innocence of the lamb, and the prudence of the serpent. She is very intelligent and gifted. She is from my native place, Charles County, and for a long time has ardently desired to be numbered among your daughters.[7]

Louisa received the name Sister Ann Simeon when she formally became a Sister of Charity. Her first mission was at the St. Peter's Orphan Asylum and Day School in Cincinnati, Ohio. Though she enjoyed teaching her students, the mission later became a trial for her.

She was recalled to Emmitsburg in 1841 and placed at the head of Saint Francis Xavier School, a school for small boys whose elder siblings were at either Mount St. Mary's or St. Joseph's. In July 1845, Sister Ann Simeon was sent to serve as Sister Servant of Saint Vincent's Asylum in Washington. It was a mission that tugged at her heart at times. Once, a child who had been neglected and left in a dirty and diseased condition came to the asylum. Sister Ann Simeon took charge of the girl, washed and cleaned her sores and cared for her until she was well.[8]

Sister Ann Simeon served at the asylum for two years before she was recalled to St. Joseph's to act as treasurer for the Sisters of Charity. As the treasurer, she also became a member of the Council of St. Joseph's, the governing body of the Sisters of Charity of St. Joseph's at Emmitsburg.

When the Sisters of Charity affiliated themselves with the Daughters of Charity in France in 1850, Sister Ann Simeon traveled with Mother Etienne Hall to Paris to learn more about their new sisters of the international community and to immerse themselves in the Vincentian spirit and tradition at the Mother House in Paris.

She was also given the duty to try and sound out the feelings of the Sisters of Charity in Cincinnati when Emmitsburg's union with France was being considered. Sister Ann Simeon interviewed each sister privately and hoped to ease the resistance the Cincinnati sisters felt toward the affiliation.

It soon became apparent that reconciliation wasn't to be and so Sister Ann Simeon returned to Emmitsburg with the sisters who chose to go back and accept the union of the two religious orders while the Sisters of Charity of Cincinnati became an independent order.[9]

This was Mother Ann Simeon's first experience with secession, but it wouldn't be her last as the war clouds began gathering over the country.

CHAPTER 5
The War Begins

"The Sisters of Charity lessened the labors of the physicians and surgeons by their humane and sympathetic labors for the welfare of thousands of suffering human beings committed to their care."

Surgeon in Chief
Lincoln Hospital

War came to the United States of America early on April 12, 1861, and with it, North and South were torn asunder.

From Fort Sumter, isolated on an island in the mouth of Charleston Harbor in South Carolina, Union troops sought to defend what they considered federal property. Just as Daniel DeLeon believed the citizens of the Confederate States owned part of the United States' medical supplies, the Confederate government believed that the funds that had paid for "federal property" had come, in part, from citizens of the Confederate States. Because of that, the Confederate government officials declared that federal property within the borders of the Confederate States would be considered part of the Confederate government.

Negotiations between the Union and Confederate governments in the months since South Carolina had seceded from the United States on December 20, 1860, had failed to find an acceptable solution.

South Carolina troops had fired on ships trying to supply Fort Sumter and turned them away, leaving the soldiers with what little rations they had in the stores. Major Robert Anderson, in command of Fort Sumter, wrote to the governor of South Carolina about the attacks, saying, "that unless it was promptly disclaimed he would regard it as an act of war, and after waiting a reasonable time he would fire upon all vessels coming within range of his guns."[1]

The shell which opened the momentous bombardment of Fort Sumter was fired at 4:30 a.m. on the morning of the April 12 from a mortar to the west of the fort from Fort Johnson on James Island. The bombardment continued for thirty-four hours until Anderson, and his men could no longer hold the fort.

General S. W. Crawford of the U.S. Army described the condition of Sumter when Anderson agreed to its surrender.

It was a scene of ruin and destruction. The quarters and barracks were in ruins. The main gates and the planking of the windows on the gorge were gone; the magazines closed and surrounded by smouldering flames and burning ashes; the provisions exhausted; much of the engineering work destroyed; and with only four barrels of powder available. The command had yielded to the inevitable. The effect of the direct shot had been to indent the walls, where the marks could be counted by hundreds, while the shells, well directed, had crushed the quarters, and, in connection with hot shot, setting them on fire, had destroyed the barracks and quarters down to the gun casemates, while the enfilading fire had prevented the service of the barbette guns, some of them comprising the most important battery in the work. The breaching fire from the columbiads and the rifle gun at Cummings point upon the right gorge's angle, had progressed sensibly and must have eventually succeeded if continued, but as yet no guns had been disabled or injured at that point. The effect of the fire upon the parapet was pronounced. The gorge, the right face and flank as well as the left face, were all taken in reverse, and a destructive fire main-

40

tained until the end, while the gun carriages on the barbette of the gorge were destroyed in the fire of the blazing
quarters.[2]

Although no one had been killed during the bombardment, as
the Union troops left the fort on April 14, a spark from a 100-gun
salute to the U.S. flag ignited a pile of cartridges. The explosion
killed Private Daniel Hough and injured other members of his
gun crew. The injured were sent to a hospital in Charleston. Private Edward Gallway died from his wounds there a few days later.

The United States was now at war with itself. American soldiers had turned on other American soldiers. Order had given
way to chaos; peace to war.

In his response to the bombardment of Fort Sumter, President
Lincoln issued a naval blockade order on April 19, 1861. It read:

For this purpose a competent force will be posted so as to
prevent entrance and exit of vessels from the ports afore-
said. If, therefore, with a view to violate such blockade, a
vessel shall approach, or shall attempt to leave either of
the said ports, she will be duly warned by the Commander
of one of the blockading vessels, who will endorse on her
register the fact and date of such warning, and if the same
vessel shall again attempt to enter or leave the blockaded
port, she will be captured and sent to the nearest
convenient port, for such proceedings against her and her
cargo as prize, as may be deemed advisable. And I hereby
proclaim and declare that if any person, under the
pretended authority of the said States, or under any other
pretense, shall molest a vessel of the United States, or the
persons or cargo on board of her, such person will be held
amenable to the laws of the United States for the
prevention and punishment of piracy.[3]

The idea behind the blockade was that if the Confederate States could not export goods, it would cut off money from commerce flowing into the Confederacy through such ports as New Orleans and Charleston.

Lincoln's plan required closing off 3,500 miles of Confederate coastline and any ports along those 3,500 miles. The blockade needed 500 ships patrolling the coast to maintain it.

Critics believed a blockade recognized the Confederate States as a nation because states in insurrection would have their ports closed not blockaded. On the other hand, under Lincoln's maritime law, a blockade gave the U.S. the right to search neutral vessels like the British that might be trying to aid the Confederate States.

At the start of the hostilities, the Daughters of Charity operated a hospital, orphanage, and school in Norfolk, Virginia. St. Mary's Asylum was a school and orphanage that the Daughters of Charity had opened in 1848. When yellow fever hit the area in 1855, eight Daughters of Charity volunteered to serve as nurses caring for the sick during that summer.

This was no small risk for the sisters. The fever eventually claimed 3,000 lives and the sisters who served among the sick were in constant danger of contracting it themselves.[4] The sisters cared for patients in their homes, in the Portsmouth Naval Hospital, in a temporary hospital four miles from Norfolk and even aboard ships. Following the epidemic, the Baltimore Steam Packet Company, which operated between Portsmouth and Baltimore, granted the Daughters of Charity free passage aboard their ships in perpetuity in gratitude for the hard for the sisters' hard work during the epidemic.[5]

More importantly, the wheels had been set in motion to open the first Catholic hospital in Virginia. Ann Behan Herron had allowed the sisters to use her home to care for patients during the yellow fever epidemic. When she died, she willed the house and grounds to the Daughters of Charity to be used as a hospital in gratitude for their service. The Daughters of Charity received the property deed and $960 a year for hospital expenses. Herron's only condition for the funds and property was that two of the wards in the hospital be reserved for charity patients.[6]

In April 1861, the Daughters of Charity serving in the Norfolk area along with the rest of the city's residents heard a train blow its shrill whistle to announce its arrival. While the train's arrival on the Norfolk and Petersburg Railroad was not surprising, the fanfare with which it announced itself was. Unknown to many in the city, the train left soon after its arrival, but the departure was done much more quietly and without any whistle blowing or loud rumbling. Shortly after that, the same train returned, again blowing its whistle often.

While residents must have wondered at the sanity of railroad owner William Mahone, Union troops across the Elizabeth River in Portsmouth thought they had something else to worry about. They believed that a huge number of Confederate troops were massing in Norfolk and that each set of whistles marked another train full of Confederate soldiers arriving into the city. This was exactly the impression Mahone wanted to create.[7]

The ruse worked. When Norfolk Navy Shipyard commander Charles Stewart McCauley heard all of the train whistles, he believed that he was facing an overwhelming Confederate force set on capturing the Union shipyard and its resources. McCauley ordered the Norfolk Naval Shipyard abandoned and destroyed, lest it fall into enemy hands.

On April 28, the Daughters of Charity hospital was emptied during the evacuation of Union troops and those residents loyal to the Union and the Marine Hospital in Portsmouth was prepared for hundreds of Union sick and wounded.

"Soon we beheld what the tolling bells had announced, the destructive fire! The Navy Yard of Portsmouth in flames! Large magazines of powder exploding shook the two cities to a fearful trembling,"[8] Sister Angela Heath wrote.

James Rada, Jr.

Union officials asked the Daughters of Charity for help in caring for the sick, and the sisters responded. "There was no time to be lost with regard to body or soul, for many we had cause to fear, had received mortal wounds in each,"[9] wrote Sister Angela. The sisters worked around the clock both in the kitchen as cooks and in the patient wards as nurses, relieving the pain and suffering of their patients. A few days after the fighting began, additional sisters arrived from the Central House in Emmitsburg to help with the nursing work. However, their trip was not without incident. "As if the enemy of souls wished to oppose their labors, they met with a delay on the road by being refused passports and again, barely escaping being lost in crossing a river in too small a boat for the number of passengers, but Divine Providence saved them,"[10] wrote Sister Angela.

The arrival of more sisters allowed those who have been there from the beginning of the fighting some relief and some frustration that the extra help hadn't come from other parties.

Many Protestant army chaplains attended these wards and some of them zealously accompanied us from bed to bed, speaking in bland tones to the dying men. "How are you, my friend? Will you have the morning paper?" "The morning paper" to a dying man, and by a minister of the Gospel![11]

Despite the hectic pace in the Portsmouth Marine Hospital, the sisters found that the soldiers appreciated their efforts. One soldier told a sister who was applying cold compresses to his fevered head, "O, if my dear mother could see your care of me, she would take heart."[12]

Even those soldiers who held a bias against Catholics found themselves moved by the tender care of the Daughters of Charity. As one soldier was brought into the hospital, he spit at the sisters when he saw them and refused to take his medicine from them.

One sister persisted in trying to get the soldier to take medicine for his own good. Finally, the soldier asked her, "Who or what are you, anyway?"

"I am a Sister of Charity," the sister replied.

"Where is your husband?"

"I have none, and I am glad I have none."

Curious, the soldier asked, "Why are you glad?"

"Because, if I had a husband, I would have to be employed in his affairs, and consequently could not be here to wait on you."

This sincere response subdued the anger in the soldier. He said, "That will do."

He turned away from the sister, but he later took his medicine and later still, he was baptized a Catholic.[13]

The Daughters of Charity spent six months in Portsmouth before the group was recalled to the Central House where they would be reassigned to a new location. During that time, their selfless service began to win them friends among those whom a year before would have scored a Catholic.

The friends of our sick soldiers at Norfolk may feel assured that every kindness and attention that can avail to comfort and cure them are ministered by the Sisters of Charity at Norfolk. The letters from the army are full of praises of these angels of mercy. We have a young friend, who probably owes his life to their unceasing watching and careful nursing. Dr. Nott, in his letter published elsewhere, writes in the same strain. A letter just received by us from a member of the 3d Alabama Regiment, says:

_____ is much better now, and is rapidly improving. I have been in to see him several times, but as the Sisters told me he was not dangerously ill. I have not written about him, for fear of causing uneasiness. He gets every attention and kindness that good nursing and medical treatment can afford. All of the soldiers have fallen in love with the Sisters for their kindness and devotion to those who are sent to their care. _____ was in their hospital for several days, and says he could not have been more tenderly and carefully nursed in his mother's house.[14]

On their way back to Emmitsburg, the train the sisters were riding on was stopped in Manassas. The Union Army was apparently firing on anyone or anything that tried to cross the Potomac River, regardless whether it was a civilian or military target.[15] The train was detoured to Richmond. Once in the Confederate capital, the sisters waited for two weeks before they could cross into the United States under a flag of truce.[16]

Richmond was a city of nearly 26,000 residents. It became the capital of the Confederate States on May 21, 1861. One of the reasons for this honor is that Richmond was the location of the Tredegar Iron Works, which produced much of the Confederate States heavy ordnance machinery.

Two days later, by a three-to-one vote, Virginia had seceded from the Union.

As the Confederate capital, Richmond would be a prize for the taking for the Union Army. So the city's defenses quickly began to take shape. They included a line of seventeen heavy batteries encircling the city about two miles out and another line of smaller batteries and trenches inside that line about a half mile out.

The inflow of soldiers and adventurers ready to fight put a strain on the city's infrastructure.

In an effort to help his efforts to care for the Confederate Army, the Confederate government had sent a telegram to the Daughters of Charity Central House in May officially requesting that sisters be specifically assigned to care for the sick and wounded Confederate soldiers in Richmond and Norfolk where they had already provided some care in the ordinary course of their nursing duties at their hospitals.

Up to this point, requests for help had always come from local military commanders. This was the first time that a government had asked the Daughters of Charity to help, but it wouldn't be the last.

Though the Daughters of Charity had proven indispensable in both New Orleans and Portsmouth, the sisters' entrance into the tense situation between the United States of America and the Confederate States of America was not met with universal approval even among the Catholic community. John Hughes, Archbishop of New York, wrote to his counterpart in Baltimore, Most Reverend Francis Patrick Kenrick, on May 9, 1861, saying:

> There is another question growing up, and it is about
> nurses for the sick and wounded. Our Sisters of Mercy
> have volunteered after the example of their Sisters toiling
> in the Crimean war. I have signified to them, not harshly,
> that they had better mind their own affairs until their ser-
> vices are needed. I am now informed indirectly that the
> Sisters of Charity in the diocese would be willing to vol-
> unteer a force of from fifty to one hundred nurses. To this
> last proposition I have very strong objections. Besides, it
> would seem to me natural and proper that the Sisters of
> Charity in Emmittsburg should occupy the very honorable
> post of nursing the sick and wounded. But, on the other
> hand, Maryland is a divided community at this moment,
> whereas New York is understood to be all on one side. In
> fact, as the question now stands, Maryland is in America,
> for the moment, as Belgium has been the battlefield of
> Europe.[17]

Still, the Daughters of Charity had a mission to seek and serve people in need. In particular, this included teaching the children and caring for the sick and dying. The war offered plenty of opportunity for the latter, and the Daughters of Charity set out to fulfill their mission.

The Daughters of Charity opened the fifty-bed Infirmary of St. Francis de Sales in Richmond. *The Richmond Dispatch* announced the opening on May 3, 1861:

> This Hospital is prepared to receive and give the best medical aid and general attention to the sick. It is a fortunate circumstance for the sick and disabled soldier stationed here that such an institution is at hand. There he will receive such nursing as no hospital not under the care of those gentle and devoted women can bestow. Let us thank God for the "Sisters of Charity," whose homes and hospitals, in the midst of wars and tumults, are an ark upon the waters, where the merciful and compassionate spirit of the Gospel, flying from the furious waves of human passions, finds a refuge till the storm be overpast.[18]

From their location on Brooke Avenue, the sisters were willing to treat any patient who didn't have a contagious disease. Though St. Francis de Sales was one of what would eventually be 140 Civil War hospitals in Richmond, within a month of its opening, it was overcrowded, sometimes holding up to 300 sick and wounded. However, the care there was considered excellent. A report in October 1861 found that from May 18 to September 23, 413 patients were treated at the hospital, and only seven had died.[19]

The St. Francis de Sales Hospital was not the only overcrowded hospital in the city. The Confederate government took over several houses and converted them into hospitals, intending that male nurses would care for the wounded.

It turned out that the men were better utilized as soldiers than caregivers. "Within a few days, the Surgeons and Officers, in charge, came to the Sisters of the Infirmary and [St. Joseph's Orphan] Asylum begging them to come to their assistance as the poor men were in much need of them," one of the sisters later wrote.[20]

It wouldn't be until the following year that the Confederate government officially recognized the superiority of female nurses over male nurses and recommended their use in hospitals. The Confederate Senate Committee on Hospitals toured many of the hospitals and made notes on the condition of the hospitals and the patients. They came away particularly impressed by nine hospitals—including St. Francis de Sales and Charity Hospital—among the dozens they visited. The shared strength among the nine hospitals was the use of female nurses. The *Richmond Enquirer* reported:

It is not alone necessary to sustain the physical being of a man by food and drink. His sympathies, his social and moral nature are of an importance, equally high, and exercise not only a controlling influence over his happiness, but, in many instances over his health. In all the qualities essential to insure these important results, it will require no power of logic in this practical and sensible age to prove that woman is greatly man's superior. Her sympathies not only soothe the afflicted, but her tenderness and kindness often afford relief. With less physical courage to resist, she yet has higher moral courage to endure, and hence, never falters or grows weary in doing good. With more heart she is necessarily more constant, more generous, more devoted and patient. - Always responsive when her humanity is appealed to, she has sympathies warmer, more religious, more earnest and refined. Her very presence is a rebuke to every impropriety, and when permanently introduced into your hospitals, will shed a gleam of neatness, cheerfulness, comfort and moral excellence around and about them not yet realized. - To the sick soldier surely nothing could be more grateful than this. In this manner, during hours of suffering, he will, to some

James Rada, Jr.

extent, realize those pure joys, which make home and
wife so dear to every manly heart, while the brave boy,
separated from friends, and prostrate upon a bed disease,
will again be reminded of her whose motherly love was
the first recollection of his childhood, and whose earnest
prayers were the first to direct his young heart to the
throne of Grace.[21]

When the Daughters of Charity had complete control over
patient care as they did at St. Francis de Sales, they could do
more for the wounded soldiers than if they worked under the direction of a physician in charge. During the time the hospital was
in operation, 2,500 soldiers were admitted. Only 100 died. This
was far less than the death rate among wounded during the war.[22]

John McGill, Bishop of Richmond, didn't mind the Daughters of Charity coming to the aid of the sick and wounded but he
did oppose them helping any hospital in competition with St.
Francis de Sales.[23]

Government officials in Richmond made requests for help
from the sisters at other hospitals, but Bishop McGill turned
them down. Finally, the sisters, realizing that they were losing an
opportunity to fulfill their mission, made their own request of
Bishop McGill. They "called at the episcopal palace and begged
to be assigned the work." In the face of such humility and a desire to serve, Bishop McGill relented.[24]

The sisters were escorted to a facility that would come to be
known as St. Ann's Military Hospital on June 26, 1861. It was so
new that the walls had yet to be plastered. The building had room
for 300 patients in wards of twelve to fourteen men.

The sisters arrived at the hospital around 10 a.m. and found
that many of the patients hadn't even eaten breakfast yet. Many
of the patients were too sick to care, but others complained of
hunger. Patients crowded the hospital filling all the bed and
many of the spaces on the floor between the beds.

The sisters went into the kitchen and found the workers earnestly trying to prepare meals. One sister wrote:

In the first place, without exaggeration, the stove might be twice as large as it is and no harm to it. Yet, to this place are stationed the regular cooks, and besides all poultice, bits of toast, boiled eggs, warmed snacks, etc., must be cooked at that stove. Imagine the place then where the nurses, sisters and cooks are all intent, upon securing their portion of the mess. Black George, when about to remove from the oven large pans of cornbread or meat will swing his arms and their contents back and forth singing out, "Clar the way, Clar the way." Then each one must look out for herself to avoid a burning.[25]

Nor did the kitchen workers have any idea about preparing meals suitable for recovering patients.[26] Many times a soldier's breakfast might be bread and coffee. The sisters set about making something more filling.

The Daughters of Charity believed in the importance of proper nutrition as part of a holistic care approach to patients. Sister Matilda Coskery wrote in her unpublished nursing guide, *Advices Concerning the Sick*:

The nurse, therefore, sh[oul]d never depart from the quantity or quality of the drinks prescribed.

The same care is necessary in point of food or nourishment – too much of the right kind w[oul]d be as bad as to give what had been objected to – If the over quantity remains undigested, he suffers much pain, and if it digest[s], it may afford to much nutriment to the system at a time when it requires less – Nothing sh[oul]d be thought small in the mind of the Nurse, where the benefit or injury of her patient is in question——

One sister arrived at the hospital later than the others. She caught up with the other Daughters of Charity in the tumultuous kitchen as they were going about preparing a meal for the soldiers. The late sister saw the pantry door wide open, so she shut and locked it. Suddenly she heard rapping on the door. "The zealous Sister was not superstitious, nor could she be called nervous, but these strong noises frightened her, and she became pale as the rappings continued to grow in volume and number."

Then the sister heard a voice asking to be let out. The sister who had shut the pantry had accidentally locked another sister inside.[27]

Despite little distractions such as this, the sisters and kitchen staff got the meal prepared and kitchen in order. The sisters were rewarded for their efforts with men who heartily enjoyed their meals, some declaring it "better than anything they had eaten since entering the army."[28] It was a first step to removing some of the discomforts among the sick soldiers.

The first night the sisters spent in the hospital was also filled with its challenges as the sick and wounded to call out either in pain or for care. The sisters responded to both needs as best they could. One of them wrote:

> We have in this hospital our brave Southern men and the
> wounded men of the North, and oh! How they suffer!
> Some of them, whose legs were amputated, were swarm-
> ing with maggots. After the dressing of one man's leg, I
> remember actually sweeping these maggots away. Yet so
> patient are the poor creatures, you seldom hear a
> complaint and they are most grateful for every little act of
> kindness.[29]

A patient who had had his leg amputated called a sister to his bedside. She came and sat in a chair next to the head of the bed. The soldier quietly said to her, "You know the doctor thinks I may not live over night, therefore, I have a great favor to ask that

I hope you will not refuse. I have a mother..."

The soldier paused as he began to weep.

"I understand. You want me to write to her," the sister said.

"Yes. Say that her child is dead, but do not tell her how I have suffered. That would break her heart."[30]

And so the Daughters of Charity began caring not just for wounded bodies but the wounded spirits of the soldiers in their care. They undoubtedly followed the advice of Sister Matilda, one of the most-experienced nurses among the Daughters of Charity.

[N]o impatience in mood or manner, they will think you give up, because you pity & feel for them, and this supposition will make them love you, and this may bring about the beginning of good deportment, and again we see the fruits of kindness, for [it] is, and forever will be, the remedy of remedies...[31]

After two weeks in Richmond, the sisters rode a train from Portsmouth north to Manassas. A Union officer boarded the train near Washington City and began walking through each rail car asking to see each passenger's identification papers to make sure spies weren't trying to make their way north. When the officer saw the Daughters of Charity, he said, "I need not question you, sisters; all is right with you. You mind your business and don't meddle with government affairs. Your society has done a great service to the country, and the authorities in Washington hold your community in high esteem."

When another officer came by later and asked to see the sisters' papers, they were more than happy to oblige, but the first officer jumped to their defense. "Let me see the man who would dare touch papers belonging to a Sister of Charity! I would give him cause to regret it," he said.

The first officer then took the papers from the sisters and wrote on them: Examined. Later, he even carried the sisters on his own boat from Fortress Monroe to Annapolis, Maryland, and chartering them a train to Baltimore from that city.[32]

In the city the sisters left, the number of hospitals in Richmond increased and the Daughters of Charity found their services requested at most of them. While they sought to fill the requests, it lessened the number of sisters at any one particular hospital.

The sisters also found conditions deteriorating as the number of wounded in the city increased. "The hospitals were often without the necessaries of life. For the Sisters' table rough corn bread and strong fat bacon were luxuries; as for beverages, they could rarely tell what was given to them for tea or coffee, for at one time it was sage and at another herbs," one historian wrote.[33]

At one of the new hospitals in Richmond where the Daughters of Charity served, the surgeon in charge told them:

Sisters, I am obliged to make known our difficulties to you, that you may enable me to surmount them, for you ladies accomplish all you undertake. Until now we have been supplied in the delicacies necessary for our patients from Louisiana, but the blockade now prevents this, and I fear to enter the wards, as the poor men are still asking for former refreshments, and they cannot be quieted. We dislike also letting them know the straits we are in, though this hindrance may be of short duration.[34]

The sisters in Richmond set out trying to figure a way to continue supplying the soldiers with the food they had grown used to. They suggested that perhaps wagons could be sent to area farmhouses to purchase things like chickens, milk, butter, fruit, and beef. The quartermaster agreed with the idea and sent the wagons out.

However, unknown to the sisters and surgeon, complaints had been made to the Confederate medical headquarters that the sisters were withholding food from the wounded soldiers. Officials sent a deputy to the hospital to investigate the charges.

[The deputy and surgeon] visited the wards during meals, after which they entered the room where the sisters dined. They then told the Surgeon the motive of their visit. He was glad to explain to them the cause of the complaints. The deputy informed the soldiers that the good sisters were not the cause of their suffering, that their fare was always worse still, then they gave to them, for when there is not enough of what is good, they take what is worse for themselves.[35]

Washington City realized the same thing as Richmond. As the Union capital, it would be a target of enemy armies. The city was younger and much less developed than Richmond. All of the government buildings had not even been completed. The Capitol Building was still without a dome. When it rained, the unpaved streets turned into a thick mud that acted like glue to wagon wheels and horses hoofs. Also, the streets were often filled with garbage.[36] Troops and artillery filled the streets and had to share it with cattle herds being driven through the city to feed the army.[37]

As Richmond had done, Washington prepared for war with a ring of fortifications around its borders and created additional medical facilities for the sick and wounded soldiers. Where the city had had only one hospital at the beginning of the war on E Street, it soon had twenty-five general hospitals in the city and surrounding suburbs with a patient capacity of more than 20,000.[38]

On June 1, 1861, Joseph Toner, a Washington physician, petitioned the sisters on behalf of a group of Washington doctors, to come build a civilian hospital in the city because the military had taken over the Washington Infirmary.[39]

The sisters accepted the offer and four of them, including Sister Sarah Carroll who was named sister servant of the group, arrived to establish Providence Hospital in a renovated mansion on

Second and D Streets in the Southeast quadrant of the city on June 10. Dr. Toner became the hospital's doctor and cared for patients at the hospital for $4 a week.

At the time, Providence was the only general hospital for civilians in a city of more than 75,000 residents and transients. The infirmary on E Street, which the Daughters of Charity had also been asked to run by local officials, had been turned into a military hospital following the fall of Fort Sumter. Though Providence Hospital was intended to be a civilian hospital, there were occasions where it was needed for military wounded as well.[40]

Mother Ann Simeon offered President Lincoln and the U.S. government the aid of the Daughters of Charity beyond Washington. The President considered the offer and asked when the sisters could start for the front. He was told that they could leave within an hour. Secretary of War Edwin Stanton sent a telegram to Emmitsburg in reply accepting the offer.[41]

The *Washington Intelligencer* reported soon after that:

> We learn that two hundred Sisters of Charity are ready to enlist in the cause of the sick and wounded of the army, at any moment the Government may signify to them a desire to avail itself of their services, to take charge of hospitals, ambulances for conveying the sick or wounded, or any post far or near, where the cause of humanity can be served.[42]

Besides the E Street Infirmary, which burned down on November 4, 1861, the Daughters of Charity were eventually asked to staff three other military hospitals in the city. Sister Camilla Bowden and eight Daughters of Charity cared for around 400 patients in the Eckington Hospital. Fourteen sisters cared for up to 1,600 wounded soldiers at a time in Cliffburne Hospital, and thirty sisters served in the Lincoln Hospital under the administration of Dr. Linsley, assistant surgeon of the U.S. Army. The hospital consisted of thirty large buildings for patients with many smaller support buildings and tents. During its four years of service, Lincoln Hospital would have more than 22,000 patients.[43]

Sister Helen Ryan became the superior of the Lincoln Hospital and the twenty-nine other Daughters of Charity there. The surgeon-in-chief would write of them, "The Sisters of Charity lessened the labors of the physicians and surgeons by their humane and sympathetic labors for the welfare of thousands of suffering human beings committed to their care."[44]

The sight of the men who had been torn apart by shrapnel, soldiers missing limbs and wrapped in bloodied bandages, men who lay in their beds moaning in pain and crying for death nearly overwhelmed the sisters, but it was a sight they would become all too familiar with. In one hospital ward, the men were skeletons of their former selves emaciated from little food and long forced marches. Few of the patients in the hospital had all their limbs.

The smell of gunpowder, rotting flesh, and bodily fluids was another thing that Civil War nurses had to overcome to work. Louisa May Alcott wrote of her first time walking into a hospital, "The first thing I met was a regiment of the vilest odors that ever assaulted the human nose, and took it by storm."[45]

Jane Grey Swisshelm, who worked as a nurse around Washington, criticized the Catholic sisters for avoiding the unpleasant work of dressing wounds.[46]

While more orders than the Daughters of Charity served in Washington, it seems highly unlikely that they would have avoided this service unless their assigned duties were elsewhere. The evidence is much greater of situations where the sisters not only dressed wounds but would occasionally perform surgery.

One such sister was Sister Anthony O'Connell, a Sister of Charity of Cincinnati, was not afraid of getting bloody. A soldier at the Battle of Shiloh wrote of her:

Amid this sea of blood she performed the most revolting duties for these poor soldiers. She seemed like a ministering angel, and many a young soldier owes his life to her

57

care and charity. Happy was the soldier who, wounded and bleeding, had her near him to whisper words of consolation and courage.[47]

On June 1, 1861, the same day Dr. Toner wrote to the Daughters of Charity Central House in Emmitsburg to ask for the sisters to nurse in Washington, Brigadier General John F. Rathbone wrote John McCloskey, Bishop of Albany, New York, to request Sisters of Charity for the more than 100 men in the military depot hospital at Albany. One sister went from St. Mary's Hospital. Rathbone had declared:

The superiority of the Sisters of Charity as nurses is known wherever the names of Florence Nightingale and the Sisters who accompanied her to the Crimea have been repeated, and these soldiers, most of whom have had woman's tender hands to minister to their want before leaving home to engage in their want before leaving home to engage in their country's battles, would feel encouraged by their kindness and care. [48]

Superiors at Emmitsburg received a telegram from Harpers Ferry on June 7 from the Confederate government, asking for Daughters of Charity to help care for the Confederate wounded in the military field hospital near Harpers Ferry.[49]

Sisters Matilda Coskery, Frances Karrer and Lucina Maher, left Emmitsburg two days later heading for Frederick, Maryland. Mother Ann Simeon had cautioned them to remain inconspicuous. The area was expecting trouble, and it would do no good for the sisters to spark it. This was a challenge since each Daughter of Charity wore the easily recognizable blue-gray dress and white cornette of a sister.

The Sisters sat as far back on the stage as they possibly could and hoped to escape observation. However, when

the stopping on a small town to change mail, the driver
threw open the coach door and passing in a letter, said:
"Sisters, here is a letter that was handed to me to give you
to mail at the first Southern Post Office after you cross the
lines!" Every eye was riveted on the Sisters but not a
question was asked.[50]

The sisters weren't aware that their destination was known,
but news travels fast and rumor even faster.

The heat of the day was the type that sucks the energy from a
person, leaving her wanting nothing more than cool shade. While
the sisters had shade in the stagecoach, it was far from cool. One
of the stagecoach horses gave out along the way and had to be
replaced, delaying the journey and leaving the sisters sweltering
in the heat themselves until another horse could be obtained.

A Confederate orderly dressed as a civilian had been sent to
escort the sisters to their destination, but they unknowingly
passed him on his way north.

In Frederick, the sisters found Union troops patrolling the
streets and camped around the edges of the city, but none interfered with the sisters or their mission. Though there was a train
depot in Frederick, the sisters couldn't use it. With Maryland and
Virginia on different sides of the war, travel on the Baltimore and
Ohio Railroad was iffy, depending on who controlled the territo-
ry south of the Potomac River. The tracks crossed from Maryland to Harpers Ferry and stayed south of the Potomac River until crossing back into Maryland near Cumberland. Whoever controlled the area could control train traffic on the Baltimore and
Ohio Railroad.

From Frederick, the Daughters of Charity were forced to continue their journey south on another stagecoach. It was a jarring
ride as the coach rolled over the rough roads. Inside, the sisters
were thrown against each other and the sides of the coach. They
were faced with a choice of either pulling the shades on the windows to try and keep out the dust being thrown up by the gallop-

ing horses and suffer the stifling heat with little air circulation or leave the shades up and choke on the dust.

The stagecoach headed southwest, and the Daughters of Charity were joined by a gentleman and lady traveling in the same direction. The oppressive heat of the day exhausted another horse that had to be replaced, once again delaying their journey. A short time later, the coach found itself stuck as it prepared to cross the Potomac River. So deeply was it mired in mud at the crossing, that it was feared the stagecoach would have to be abandoned. The men did finally manage to free the vehicle, and the journey continued.

After passing through the Union camp posts, it was near twilight when they met their first Southern picket.

> Each picket haled the carriage and asked the intentions of the passengers. The gentleman replied: "These ladies are coming to serve your sick men; this lady and I are Southerners returning to Richmond, Virginia." The Sisters were permitted to pass on, but at each post there was the same interrogatory. The last picket, however, held them until the Officer in command should come.[51]

The same questions were once again asked and the same answers were given. The officer allowed them to pass, but he crossed the Potomac River bridge with them over "kegs of powder were placed here and there so that in case the Northern Army approached, it could be instantly blown up." [52]

They arrived at the Harpers Ferry military hospital, which was on a hill high above the town and bounded by the two rivers. The hospital was filled with sick and wounded, and Sister Matilda estimated there were 40,000 to 50,000 troops in town when they arrived.[53]

Situated at the confluence of the Potomac River and Shenandoah River, the small town was not only a stop on the Baltimore and Ohio Railroad, but it was just across the river from the Chesapeake and Ohio Canal in Maryland. This made it a strategic location to have troops stationed who could be deployed along the rail line or cross into Maryland to stop traffic on the canal. Until just a few months earlier, it had been the location of the United States Arsenal and Armory and Hall's Rifle Works.

Most of Harpers Ferry's residents had supported the Union during Virginia's secession debate. The superintendent of the armory, Alfred Barbour had supported the Confederacy, however. He told the armory employees that the arsenal would be turned over to Confederate forces. Lieutenant John Rogers believed otherwise, and he had set fire to the buildings to keep them from falling into Confederate hands the day after Virginia voted to secede from the Union.

Major General Kenton Harper had brought the Virginia militia to occupy the town until Colonel Thomas J. Jackson arrived on April 27, 1861. He organized the militia and salvaged what he could from the arsenal ruins to ship to Richmond. He also began fortifying the town.

General Joseph E. Johnston took over command on May 24, 1861. Despite the fortifications, he believed the town made too easy a target for artillery that could be positioned on the higher surrounding mountains, particularly those on the Maryland side of the Potomac River.

Despite the heat during the sisters' journey, a cold spell had passed through Harpers Ferry earlier making many of the soldiers sicker than they already were. Many were forced to lay suffering in their own tents until beds opened up in the hospital or in private homes. Sister Matilda wrote, "The men in one regiment had contracted measles on their march; this spreading among others with exposure incidental to army life thinned their numbers before the ball and sword had begun their quicker work."[54]

The sisters quickly learned that poor hygiene was just as great an enemy to the soldiers as an opposing army. The Daughters of Charity believed, "Every thing disgusting smell or sight must be removed as soon as possible."[55] Patients needed fresh

61

air. They needed to be clean. They needed fresh food that could be eaten with clean utensils. They needed to be cleaned when they soiled themselves.

This wasn't happening at Harpers Ferry, and the sisters saw the results. Many men had been cared for by mothers and wives and once on their own, neglected washing themselves and their clothes. They ignored camp sanitation, inviting odors, flies, and disease into their camps.

It hadn't taken long for the men to sicken. The most common symptom was diarrhea, which marked the onset of dysentery, tuberculosis, and malaria.

The silence during their first night with so many thousands of soldiers nearby was unsettling to the sisters, but Harpers Ferry was a town that lived in fear. "Not a light gleamed from the fastened windows for fear of discovery by the hidden enemy. The whole army had been sleeping or resting on their arms since their arrival, expecting an early attack," Sister Matilda wrote.[56]

The medical director for Harpers Ferry escorted the sisters to the main hospital atop Bolivar Heights in the morning. The entire town had, in essence, been turned into a hospital. Churches and mills had become hospitals wards while shops and residences had become barracks and stables.

As the medical director and his assistant took the sisters through the buildings and the various wards, they introduced the women to the soldiers and said, "Now you will have no cause to complain of not getting nourishment, medicine and attention at the right time, for the Sisters of Charity will see to all these thi[n]gs."[57]

Not only did camp cooking leave a lot to be desired, but it was poor in nutrition. Fresh fruits and vegetables were rare, particularly when the army was on the march. Generally, the meals consisted of preserved beef, salt pork, beans, coffee, and hardtack. The surrounding countryside did not prove to be a source of food, either. Both the Union and Confederate armies had occupied the area, so it was "completely drained of provisions, necessary conveniences for the sick, etc., so that the poor sick and all around them had much to suffer."[58]

Before the sisters could get to work helping in the hospital and making a difference for the soldiers, a telegram arrived ordering the Confederate Army to Winchester, Virginia. The Union Army was expected to cross the Potomac River, above and below Harpers Ferry, in an attempt to capture the town. The Confederate Army was in no condition to defend itself, so it needed to withdraw from the town.

Soldiers destroyed their tents and provisions, burned bridges and tore up the rail tracks to leave nothing behind for the enemy to use. Then they began a mass evacuation of all of the sick and wounded.

Sister Matilda wrote about how the destruction continued through the night.

Arrangements are now being made for the several explosions and we were sent to remain with a worthy Catholic family further from these buildings. During the night, one after another, the Grand Bridge in its turn shook heights, valley, and town. The little Church (Catholic), the only one that had not been applied to military purposes, was filled and surrounded by the frightened people.[59]

The following day the sisters waited, expecting a messenger to tell them when they could board a rail car to Winchester. Sister Matilda wrote:

We now heard the Ladies of Winchester had written to the Medical Director "not to have the Sisters of Charity serve the sick, that they [the ladies] would wait on them." … They [the physicians] said; "No, they cared nothing for the objections that had been made to them on that matter; that those Ladies could never do for the sick as the Sisters of Charity would do, and therefore, unless we insisted on

63

returning home [to Emmitsburg], they held us to our undertaking."[60]

Local women could be frustrating in other ways as well. Unlike the Catholic sisters who treated everyone the same regardless of which side they fought on, town women could be very discriminating in their aid. Harriet Dada, a Civil War nurse, noted that in a hospital where she worked, Confederate women would bring things to comfort the Confederate wounded but ignored the Union wounded in the hospital. Finally, the Confederate surgeon in charge had to tell the women they wouldn't be allowed in the hospital if they kept up their bias toward the wounded.[61]

The sisters waited to hear word of when they would board the train to Winchester. No notice came and around 11 p.m., they started to get ready for bed. That's when the woman of the house came to their room and said, "My dear, poor Sisters, a wagon and your baggage are at the door for you."[62]

The sisters quickly dressed and boarded the wagon. Two black men drove them through the cloudy night with only an occasional star seen. The pastor of the Catholic church in Harpers Ferry, Rev. Michael Costello, traveled with them to watch over the sisters.

They reached the depot in town, and the pastor led them across a temporary bridge, nothing more than two planks across the water, to a shelter where they could wait for the train.

The Confederate train arrived before dawn, traveling on the tracks of the B&O Railroad. The journey to Winchester by train took five hours with the wounded crammed together uncomfortably the entire time.

Disembarking from the train, the Daughters of Charity looked at the thousands of men lying on the ground waiting to be taken to a hospital, the sisters realized that there were too many soldiers for the four sisters to care for.[63] The sisters also found themselves without a place to stay because all of the available rooms were understandably filled with sick and wounded soldiers. Father Costello took them to a local church to wait while he went off in search of lodgings.

The sight of the sisters walking through the town attracted a crowd who followed them to the church. Some of the more curious townspeople even crept into the church and sneaked peeks through the cracks in the confessionals to look at the sisters.[64]

The women waited patiently until the next day for someone to come and inform them where they would be needed. Tired of doing nothing, the sisters left the room and finally began their work in the largest hospital in Winchester. They were nearly overwhelmed by the tasks of caring for all of the sick and wounded soldiers. They dressed wounds as best they could, but other men needed the attention of a surgeon, and the sisters could do little to bring them comfort, though they tried.

In need of additional help that the Confederate government couldn't supply, the sisters decided that one of them should return to Emmitsburg and bring back additional aid.

Sister Matilda expressed her willingness to face the perilous journey alone. With a scant supply of food, she set out placing her sole trust in God who was about to confirm sweetly in her case, His promise never to permit those who trust in Him to be confounded.

Sister Matilda crossed the Potomac River in a flatboat. Landing on the Maryland side, she had to hurry by foot over a mile to catch the Northern train. The railroad officials, unwilling to take anyone across the lines, threatened to put her off at the nearest station."[65]

She reached Frederick that night quite exhausted. She slept in town and took the next stagecoach north in the morning, arriving that evening to a relieved community who worried that they hadn't heard a word from the sisters.

Upon hearing Sister Matilda's report, Sister Valentine Latour-aduais, sister servant of Saint Mary's Asylum in Saint Louis, was summoned by telegraph to relieve Sister Matilda at Winchester. Three other sisters were sent south to help in Win-

James Rada, Jr.

chester as well.

Sister Euphemia Blenkinsop and three sisters were also dispatched to Richmond where their services were needed.

CHAPTER 6
Spilled Blood

"We were for two long days in the very midst of the sounds of war...our poor sisters, though the shells were flying around them, did not even interrupt their duties....The soldiers asked one another: 'How is it that the sisters do not tremble? As for us, we are used to the noises of cannon and shells, but they are very different, and yet they go about as if nothing were the matter.' Others asked the sisters what we should do if the enemy should reach us in triumph! 'We should remain at our post.'"

Sister Euphemia Blenkinsop
Daughter of Charity

Though there had been fighting between the Union and Confederate armies in early 1861, the two hadn't yet met on the ground in a battle that would cause significant casualties.

That soon changed.

In July 1861, men began gathering near the Manassas, Virginia, railroad junction.

Brigadier General Irvin McDowell commanded the Army of Northeastern Virginia for the Union. Almost from the date of his appointment, he not only had to deal with training his inexperienced army but also with placating impatient politicians and Washington residents who wanted a quick and decisive victory over the Confederate Army, particularly after the loss of Fort

Sumter in South Carolina. On July 16, 1861, McDowell left Washington with his army of 35,000 men.

The Confederate Army of the Potomac was smaller with only 22,000 soldiers who were just as untrained as their counterparts in the Union Army. Brigadier General P. G. T. Beauregard had the army camped at Manassas Junction about twenty-five miles from the nation's capital.

McDowell planned to overwhelm Beauregard with his vastly larger army. He aimed his attack at his enemy's flank, but Beauregard recognized McDowell's intentions and moved to meet the attack on their left flank. The Confederate Army was also able to build up troop strength on the Union right side and overrun that flank.

The resulting rout of the Union Army sent soldiers scrambling in a disorderly retreat back to Washington City. The Federals suffered about 2,952 casualties (killed, wounded, and captured or missing), and the Confederates had about 1,752 casualties.

One of the reasons for the high number of casualties throughout the war was the medical care the soldiers received. The knowledge of what was a good medical practice was evolving. Just as actually working with sick and afflicted patients in hospitals and during public health crises helped the Daughters of Charity improve their skills and practices, so too, would the Civil War improve medicine in general, but first doctors and nurses would have to see what wasn't working.

One controversial treatment, even among doctors, was amputations. Some felt that given the high chances of infections from lying on the battlefield with open wounds that amputations saved lives. Other doctors reluctantly felt that, although a limb might have been saved if the doctor had had plenty of time to work on it, it just wasn't possible under battlefield conditions when thousands of soldiers needed treatment.

Dr. William Keen wrote of his wartime experiences with the benefit of years of hindsight saying:

We operated in our old blood-stained and often pus-stained coats....We used undisinfected instruments from undisinfected plush cases, and still worse, used marine sponges which had been used in prior pus cases and had been only washed in tap water. If a sponge or instrument fell on the floor it was washed and squeezed in a basin of tap water and used as if it were clean. ... The silk with which we sewed up all our wounds was undisinfected. If there was any difficulty in threading the needle we moistened it with (as we now know) bacteria-laden saliva, and rolled it between our bacteria-infected fingers. ...In opening wounds...maggots as large as chestnut worms abounded in the Summer. While disgusting they did little or no harm.[1]

In Sister Matilda's *Advices Concerning the Sick*, she wrote, "All the vessels used for medicines, drinks or nourishment, sh[oul]d be cleansed the instant they are used; consequently, the same vessel or spoon shop[oul]d not be used twice without its being cleaned, or used for two persons without washing."[2] It is not a leap to believe that had Sister Matilda been writing of surgery, she would have advised similar measures. The sisters worked to introduce such practical nursing skills wherever they served.

Providence Hospital in Washington had only been operating for six weeks when the armies clashed at Manassas. Sister Lucy Gwynn, sister servant at St. Vincent's Orphanage, negotiated with the doctors on how this new civilian hospital would be run. The Nicholson Mansion, at the corner of Second and D streets, was rented from the widow of the quartermaster general of the Marine Corps, Sarah Carroll Nicholson.[3]

Though planned as a civilian hospital, Providence Hospital, as well as most of the larger buildings in the city, were about to become military hospitals.

The Union Army had no method for getting the wounded off the battlefield, and in the confusion of the rout by the Confederates, many of the injured found themselves forced to walk the twenty miles back to Washington City. Some of the wounded checked themselves into the Willard Hotel in Washington and sought help from local doctors.[4]

Getting the wounded off the battlefields in order for them to receive care could be almost as painful for a wounded man as when he was shot. Farm wagons with no springs and horses were confiscated from nearby farms to be used as ambulances. The wounded were laid in the wagon bed and bounced against the hard wood while the driver hurried to get the wounded to a battlefield hospital or first aid station. There, they might be given emergency surgery to stabilize their condition only to have to endure more jarring bouncing over rutted roads to get to a hospital for long-term care.[5]

This is not to say that the army didn't have ambulance wagons, but the drivers wouldn't take orders from the doctors because the ambulance corps was under the direction of the quartermasters.

The ambulances that poured into Washington with the retreating army held drivers, officers, soldiers, even civilians, but very rarely carried a wounded man. Many doctors, fled, abandoning all pretense at treating the wounded. Others stayed behind and were taken prisoners by the rebels.[6]

This problem of keeping a soldier alive so that he could be transported to a hospital led to the development of battlefield hospitals. They were temporary treatment areas where wounded soldiers got their first help after a battle. It would also expand the opportunities for the Daughters of Charity to serve where they could be even more useful.

Following the rout at Manassas, casualties poured into Washington on flatbed cars and steamers through the ports of Alexandria and Georgetown. They were carried to hospitals so overcrowded that orderlies began laying them outside in tent hospitals that ranged from the Capitol to Providence Hospital. Capitol Hill became known as "bloody hill."[7]

Further South, in Richmond, the first trains arriving from the battlefield carried only the mildly wounded or those who had been incapacitated by marching. These men traveled sitting in the passenger cars. But the trains continued to arrive all day Monday and into the evening, and the injuries grew worse with each new train. The black smoke from the engine stacks came to symbolize that death was arriving in the town. The later trains carried the most-seriously injured soldiers lying on flatbed cars without anyone to give them care or attention. Many of the wounds had received no treatment. Pus mixed with dirt and formed a crust that held the bandages in place. Many of the men had had nothing to eat or drink during the long journey.

Each train seemed to carry more horribly wounded soldiers, those hardest to evacuate from the field of battle. No one knew if this train bore the final contingent of the seriously wounded, or if another train would soon arrive, bringing soldiers even more terribly mangled.[8]

Confederate Surgeon General Daniel DeLeon's hospitals were soon overflowing with wounded soldiers and private citizens began to take soldiers into their homes as adopted members of their families. Though compassionate, these civilians and even few of the actual doctors and surgeons in the area were used to seeing such damage done to the human body. Chief Nurse Abby Gibbons wrote after a battle near Winchester in 1862:

There are about 20 of the wounded ones who, I think, must die; and many of them, because of the unskillful [sic] and positively ignorant butchery of many calling themselves surgeons. Oh, it is too sad, to see fine men sacrificed, whose lives might have been saved.[9]

James Rada, Jr.

Soldiers observed the surgery performed on others, or upon themselves, and could not help but note the similarity: "It was butchery, sheer butchery, pure butchery," is the comment of a hundred diaries. The surgery was performed in one large room in the house, or in the center of the barn, or in an open tent, or on a table under the open skies, but surgery always occurred with many people watching. Doctors watched to learn; officers watched with a strange and somewhat perverse fascination; all sorts of passersby stopped for a moment to observe. The most pitiable class of observers were those who were waiting in line to lose their own limbs.[10]

To try and accommodate the wounded, the Confederate authorities moved many of the sick to larger quarters outside of the city. The government took over mansions and converted them into hospitals. Other wounded soldiers were sent out on trains to other cities such as Charlottesville, Virginia.

The Daughters of Charity hadn't been asked to help with the new hospitals, so they continued their work at St. Francis de Sales Infirmary. On July 26, 1861, Dr. Charles Bell Gibson, facing the overwhelming number of wounded coming into town from Manassas, requested that the sisters help care for the wounded at St. Ann's Military Hospital, Richmond. Eight Daughters of Charity arrived in the city to nurse the sick and wounded in an unfinished building constructed as an Alms House. Each room became a ward for twelve to fourteen men. In all, the eight sisters had about 300 soldiers to care for.

The second night the Sisters were there fifty wounded soldiers and prisoners from Manassas were brought in and placed on the hospital floor. In order to dress the patients' wounds, the Sisters had to cut away infected flesh because the soldiers had lain on the battlefield several days. They also got cots and clothing for their patients. When more wounded arrived, Sisters from the asylum and in-

72

firmary helped out also.[11]

During the battle, it was said that the sisters could almost hear the reverberating shot and shell from the fight, though it was ninety miles away. The sisters worked tirelessly, treating both Union and Confederate wounded with the same attention and care. Sister Euphemia described the work and care the Daughters of Charity provided in Richmond:

It is very extensive, and consequently requires a great deal of time for the service. Besides preparing the remedies, the Sisters are entrusted with the clothes-room, the superintendence of the kitchen, distribution of wine, etc. They are nearly always obliged to cleanse and dress the patients' wounds themselves, for otherwise they would be forgotten. There is so much suffering and so much to be done.[12]

In one hospital, a doctor called to one sister, "Sister, get something for this poor man's head. He has just asked for a piece of wood."

The sister searched for an available pillow but couldn't find one. Finally, she did find an empty pillowcase and had the idea to stuff it with paper. She brought it to the soldier, who was a wounded Union soldier. He took the pillow with a smile.[13]

The sisters all worked a long day that exhausted them. While one would expect them to fall asleep quickly after such a day, they didn't.

"I cannot sleep; there is such an odor of death about this apartment," Sister Blanche Rooney remarked.

They managed as best they could and in the morning, they found the cause of the odor. A pair of amputated limbs had been carelessly thrown into another room. Sister Blanche covered her mouth with a handkerchief and rushed into the room long enough to open a window. Soon after that, she gave directions to have the limbs interred.

"Yesterday a man was buried with three legs," she wrote in her diary.[14]

On the day of the Battle of Manassas, eleven Union officers were added to the number of patients at the hospital. Because of the crowded conditions in the hospital and their rank, they were given a room in the garret near where the sisters' room was located.

One of the officers was loaned a guitar, and he spent much of his time singing and playing the instrument. The music attracted many curious spectators who watched the Union officers and asked questions. Some of the officers became annoyed with answering the same questions over and over.

"Where were you shot at?" one person asked one of the officers.

While the questioner wanted to know where on his body the officer was wounded, the man replied, "Shot at Manassas."[15]

Once one of the officers asked said to one of the sisters, "You ladies have a sight of work to do, but I tell you what, you get high pay."

"None at all," the sister quietly replied.

"What? You don't tell me you do all this work for nothing?"

"Precisely."

The Union officers would remember that, and later five of them would send the sisters a check for fifty dollars to benefit their orphanage in Richmond.[16]

The sisters also continued their work with patients further east in Norfolk. A soldier with the Third Alabama Regiment wrote a letter to the newspapers, talking about the treatment of a fellow Confederate soldier by the Daughters of Charity, saying, "He gets every attention and kindness that good nursing and medical treatment can afford. All of the soldiers have fallen in love with the Sisters for their kindness and devotion to those who are sent to their care. _____ was in their hospital for several days, and says he could not have been more tenderly and carefully nursed in his mother's house."[17]

The *Charleston Mercury* wrote about the work of the Daughters of Charity in the Southern hospitals:

... Thus one passes on from bed to bed through the many wards, and reads the awful moral of this unholy war in the saddest illustrations which the vices and passions of men can furnish. And yet, through all this gloom and suffering, a gleam of light shoots like a golden thread on a funeral pall. I have told you how clean and neat the rooms are, and how comfortable the patients look. And the secret of the pleasant fact lies in that woman flitting across the corridor, with her gray serge dress and tidy blue apron from chin to toe, and bonnet blanc, whose wide flaps, white as a snow drift, and stiff with starch, wave over her shoulders like a pair of wings. She is one of that devoted band of good women, known all over the Christian world wherever there is sorrow to be assuaged, or pain relieved, or comfort administered, whom we name "Sisters of Charity," but who should be called the "Angels of the Earth." Her step is swift-paced and noiseless, her hand light and soft, her care and attention devoted, unobtrusive, intelligent, gentle and consoling. She it is on whom these grave, thoughtful surgeons lean, to support and carry out all their directions for the sick; and these miserable men to lighten the burden of their pain and captivity. If a biscuit or a mattress, a cup of water, a clean pillow or fresh bed or body clothes are wanted, the universal demand which satisfies every desire is, "Call a Sister!" Day and night, with tireless patience; kind, considerate and obliging to all alike; asking no recompense and accepting no reward, their skilful (sic) ministrations are bestowed on these wounded enemies, whose malignant hate and unspeakable purposes of rapine and violence to their sex (had victory crowned their arms), they are now repaying with a care and gentleness "mild as any mother's to a sick child." With such a reality before us, we may well pass by with contempt and scorn the foul charges of cruelty which the Northern press has falsely laid upon us, and retort upon them their own inhumanity and unchristian neglect in neither tending their wounded nor securing decent burial for their dead . . .[18]

In the border state of Missouri, the need for medical care was growing because of the war. On August 12, 1861, Union Major General John C. Fremont "desired that every attention be paid to soldiers who had exposed their lives for their country, visited them frequently, and believing that there was much neglect on the part of the attendants, applied to the Sisters at St. Philomena's School, St. Louis, for a sufficient number of sisters to take charge of the hospital, promising to leave everything to their management."[19] Because of the reputation of the Daughters of Charity, he promised he would leave the management of the hospital as well as the care of the sick and wounded in the hands of the sisters.

On a visit to St. Philomena's School earlier in the year Father Burlando and Mother Ann Simeon had foreseen the possibility of such a need arising and left directions for how the sisters in Missouri should handle the request when the time arose. They enacted those directions at this time.

Twelve sisters from St. Philomena's went to the Military Hospital House of Refuge in the suburbs of St. Louis. The sisters took charge of the hundreds of patients in the wards and whatever related to the sick and wounded. Peter Kenrick, Archbishop of St. Louis, sent a chaplain to say daily Mass for them. It soon became the primary location to send wounded Confederate POWs who were brought up the Mississippi River on hospital steamboats. The Union wounded were sent to City Hospital.[20]

At first, the sisters were a wonder to behold because of their strange dress and some patients asked them if they were Freemasons.[21] The patients were grateful for the fine care they received, and because of that, they gave the sisters their respect and cooperation. Women from the Union Aid Society visited the soldiers every other day. These women grew to admire the peace that reigned in the wards overseen by the Daughters of Charity and found the patients "as submissive as children."[22]

Often when the soldiers returned to their regiments, they told other sick or wounded soldiers, "If you go to St. Louis, try to get to the House of Refuge Hospital. The Sisters are there, they will make you well soon."[23]

Sisters from St. Louis also visited Jefferson Barracks Hospital, nine miles from the city.[24] The primary duty of the military camp would shift from training soldiers to saving their lives by 1862. As a hospital, the barracks had over 3,000 beds.[25]

A sister on her nightly rounds came upon a soldier whose hand had been amputated. The man was suffering, and his arm looked bright red and swollen. The soldier told the sister that a doctor had ordered a hot poultice for his arm that morning, but he hadn't received it.

The sister found a nurse and asked why the doctor's orders had been ignored. The nurse told her that there were no hops in the hospital with which to make the poultice. The hospital steward had gone into town for supplies that morning before it was known that hops were needed and there had been no other opportunity to send someone else into town.

The sister went across the yard to another building and got hops from a bakery that was nearby. She then had the poultice made.

The man said once he got relief, "The Sisters find ways and means to relieve everyone, but others who make a profession of the work do not even know how to begin it."[26]

The Daughters of Charity primary purpose during the war was to serve as nurses, but their selfless work bore fruit that helped them further their religious mission as well. It is believed that there were more baptisms in the House of Refuge Military

James Rada, Jr.

Hospital than in any of the hospitals or on the battlefield during the Civil War. Estimates are that that between 500 and 600 people were baptized at the hospital.[27]

In one such instance, a young soldier who was a Methodist was brought into the hospital in a weakened state. The doctors examined him and said he had no hope for recovery, yet the sisters continued to give him their care.

"If I had been brought here when I was first taken sick and had you sisters to take care of me, I would have been cured long ago," the soldier told one of the sisters.

The soldier's condition continued to deteriorate. One evening a sister slid a Medal of Our Blessed Mother under the soldier's pillow and prayed for him.

A few hours later, an excited nurse rushed in to find the sister. "Come quickly and see the man who died and came back to life again," the woman said.

The sister followed the nurse to the bed of the Methodist soldier to find him no longer near death. [28]

Father John Patrick Ryan saw one example of how the Catholic sisters affected the spirits of the soldiers they aided. His story began before the war in Boston. A sister walking on the street was so rudely addressed by a young man that her cheeks flushed.

Fast forward to the war, a wounded Union soldier at the St. Louis Military Hospital realized he was dying from his injuries. A sister working in the hospital asked the man to be baptized and confess his sins.

The soldier told her, "I have committed many sins in my life, and I am sorry for them all and hope to be forgiven; but there is one thing that weighs heavy on my mind at this moment. I once insulted a Sister of Charity in the streets of Boston. Her glance of reproach has haunted me ever since. I know nothing of the sisters then. But now I know how good and disinterested you are and how mean I was. Oh! If that sister were only here, weak and dying as I am, I would go down upon my knees and ask her pardon."

"If that is all you desire to set your mind at ease, you can have it," the sister said. "I am the sister you insulted, and I grant you pardon freely and from my heart."

The soldier's eyes widened. "What! Are you the sister I met in Boston? Oh, yes, you are – I know you now. And how could you have attended on me with greater care than on any of the other patients? – me, who insulted you."

The humble sister nodded. "It is the Lord's way. I did it for His Sake, because He loved His enemies and blessed those who persecuted Him. I knew you from the moment you entered the hospital. I recognized you from the scar over your forehead, and I have prayed for you unceasingly."

"Send for the priest," the soldier told her. "The religion that teaches such charity must be from God."

By the time death finally took him, the soldier had been baptized. He died murmuring a prayer the sister had taught him.[29]

Though President Lincoln prohibited all trade with the Confederate States, on August 16, 1861, a group of nine sisters left Emmitsburg on August 21 and were able to reach Richmond four days later. This band of sisters traveled by military permit and under military escort.[30]

Daughters of Charity already in the South were dispatched to Pensacola, Florida, to the Marine Hospital between the Confederate Navy Yard and Fort Barrancas. The *Charleston Mercury* noted that sisters were in charge of the facility. Six had been sent from Mobile, Alabama, and three had been sent from New Orleans.[31]

In September, the Confederates were again sending their wounded soldiers to St. Francis de Sales Infirmary in Richmond.[32] The work of the sisters had already been noticed and was appreciated by the city's residents. The *Richmond Dispatch* noted:

The world-wide benevolence of that revered order, the Sisters of Charity, meets in our city with an ample field for its exercise. The casualties of the battle-field, not less than the diseases incident to those unaccustomed to the hardships of camp life, all contribute to swell the catalogue of human ills, and leave in our midst objects of their attention, not less of the enemy than our own. Where sickness and death visit the hospitals, where are congregated the weary, wounded and dying, there, gliding in to succor and console, the sisters came upon their errand of mercy. The couch of disease is made easier by their presence; the pillow of the dying is smoothed by their care; friend and enemy alike receive their soothing attentions.--Worldly fame they ask not. Unobtrusive in their charities as in their garb, they engage in their labor of love, actuated by that pure philanthropy which has its source in a higher sphere than earth. The task imposed upon themselves, and faithfully executed by these self-sacrificing women, sometimes "even unto death," should entitle them to the rewards of the blessed. Some of those now in our midst came from Washington, by stealth, after in vain soliciting from the petty tyrant who reigns there, permission to pass the bounds of his army; some came from the far South. Come, however, from where they may, they all act as ministering angels, actuated alone by the desire to do good.[33]

As it seemed that the sisters would be performing a lot of nursing during the conflict, Father Burlando issued a list of conditions that needed to be met for the Daughters of Charity to serve on either side of the conflict.

1. "That no lady volunteers be associated with the Sisters in the duties as such an association would be rather an encumbrance than a help."

2. "That the Sisters should have entire charge of the hospitals or ambulances."

3. "That the government pay the travelling expenses of the

Sisters and furnish their board and other actual necessities during the war-clothing also in case it should be protracted."

4. "That a Catholic chaplain be in attendance."[34]

Also, Father Burlando sent a twelve-page letter of instructions to the sisters at the military hospitals about their conduct toward their patients and observance of their religious duties. He recommended the virtues of humility, modesty, and charity. "The work which you are engaged in is God's own work, the poor sufferers whom you are endeavoring to relieve are God's own children and are you not also the cherished children of God."[35] He pointed out that it was necessary to be faithful to their spiritual exercises. If they must omit them, they should get permission to do so.

> When you bandage a wounded foot or hand, think of the
> Sacred hands and feet of our Lord pierced by the sharp
> nails, when you smooth the pillow under the head of the
> dying soldier, think of the agonizing head of your
> Redeemer, then you may justly hope that these will be
> genuine Acts of Charity.[36]

He also cautioned them about their words and personal feelings about the fighting.

> For some months past you have no doubt, anxiously
> viewed the gathering storm which is threatening the
> beautiful horizon of our Country -- you are aware of the
> conflicting opinions which disturb the peace of our Cities
> & distract the minds of our Citizens -- Friend is armed
> against friend, & brothers, Fathers, & Sons enlist on
> opposite sides, in the struggle -- Our once happy land is
> plunged in anarchy & confusion, & deluged with the
> blood of its own sons.
> In this sad & lamentable state of things, I think it duty
> to remind you, my dear Sisters of the maxim of St.

James Rada, Jr.

Vincent, which was, to refrain from uttering Political sentiments - this judicious silence he left to his children as a legacy after his death as he had practiced & warmly recommended it during life -- You, as his devoted Daughters understand the obligation of adhering strictly to the wise lessons he gave you, & consequently, you will carefully abstain from speaking or writing about political affairs of our Country - It is not the sphere of the Daughters of St. Vincent to discourse about Politics of which they are, & should be uninformed - Their only duty is to sanctify themselves in the Exercise of charity according to their Rules; they leave State affairs to God & to those entrusted with them - They have no Enemy but pride & the evil spirit - North, South, East or West are alike to them; every afflicted member of society is their friend & an object of their Solicitude, because he represents their suffering Saviour, the Immaculate Spouse of their soul & the great pattern of charity whom they should strive to imitate especially by the performance of deeds of charity wherever holy obedience sends them. This is their particular duty, their noble mission, their life, their existence.[37]

In October, Sister Regina, who still managed the sisters in New Orleans, sent three of them from Charity Hospital and one sister from the Infant Asylum to nurse sick Confederate soldiers at Holly Springs, Mississippi, as the fighting continued.[38]

CHAPTER 7
Sister Euphemia "The Little Saint"

*"Are the Sisters of Charity really better nurses
than most other women?" I asked an intelligent
lady who had seen much of our military hospitals.
"Yes they are," was her reply. "Why should it be
so?" "I think it is because with them it is a work
of self-abnegation, and of duty to God, and they
are so quiet and self-forgetful in its exercise that
they do it better, while many other women show
such self-consciousness and are so fussy!"*

*Catherine Ester Beecher &
Harriet Beecher Stowe*

With the fighting between the Union and the Confederacy now at the level of an all-out war, the Daughters of Charity, who had been able to move with relative ease between North and South and back again, were having trouble communicating with their sisters in distant cities in the South.

Owing to the difficulties of communication between the
Sisters in the South and the Superior of the Central
House, it was decided necessary to send some one author-
ized to represent the Visitatrix in the states. Therefore, the
Council was unanimous in selecting, Sister Euphemia
[Blenkinsop], Assistant, for that mission.[1]

Sister Euphemia was fifty-five years old at the time when she was named the Daughters of Charity Visitatrix to the Confeder-

83

ate States on November 2, 1861. She had been born Catherine Blenkinsop in Dublin, Ireland on April 4, 1816, and lived the first ten years of her life in Dublin. She had been a sister since she was fifteen years old.

In 1826, her parents and their five children had come to America to make a better life for themselves. Between 1820 and 1830 nearly 4.5 million Irish immigrated to America, accounting for nearly a third of all the country's immigrants.[2] One of the common ports of entry was Baltimore, Maryland, behind only New York City and Boston as the most-common port of entry for Europeans. And so, the Blenkinsops found themselves coming ashore in their new country at Baltimore City.

Most of the Irish immigrants had left behind a rural life on the Emerald Isle, and they now found themselves in crowded cities. Though not considered poor in their homeland, they were destitute in America. They crowded into living spaces with single-family homes often subdivided to hold many more families. Inadequate sewage and lack of adequate running water made cleanliness that much harder and allowed disease to run rampant.

Because a good number of Irish immigrants were farmers, they lacked the skills needed to live in a city with any degree of prosperity. Many became laborers.

Peter Blenkinsop, Catherine's father, was lucky in that he had skills useful in a city. He established himself as a bookseller in Baltimore and, among other things, would publish *Metropolitan*, the city's first monthly Catholic magazine.

The Blenkinsops gave all of their children to the Catholic Church. This is not surprising since Mrs. Blenkinsop was the sister of Archbishop Oliver Kelly of Tuon.[3] Catherine's two brothers, William and Peter, both became priests, and Catherine became a Sister of Charity.

Even as a young girl, Catherine had a piety and innocence that earned her the nickname, "the little saint." In one instance, she discovered a woman of the parish was not attending Mass because she did not want to leave her children alone with their nurse and the household servants. Catherine gained the woman's confidence to the point where the woman returned to church, leaving the children in Catherine's care.[4]

One of Catherine's first·friends upon arriving in Baltimore was not another young girl or boy but a Sulpician priest, Father Louis Deluol.[5] He recognized the spiritual qualities in Catherine's nature and directed her toward the Sisters of Charity. She applied for entrance in April 1831 at the age of fifteen.

Once accepted, she was anxious to be off to Emmitsburg and begin her religious formation for service to persons who were poor. Father Deluol was preparing to visit the sisters in Emmitsburg when he stopped in to say goodbye to Catherine and her family.

Half in jest, he said, "Katie, I am going to Saint Joseph's. Would you like to come with me?"

"Oh, yes, Father!" was her immediate answer.

"But, child, you are not ready!"

"I can get ready in a few minutes, Father, if you will only take me."[6]

She rushed off to find her parents and ask their permission. The Blenkinsops agreed, and so, Catherine traveled to Emmitsburg and entered the sisterhood on May 6, 1831. She received the name Euphemia – which means harmonious and agreeable – when she donned the religious habit.

Sister Euphemia's first mission was to St. Joseph's School in New York City, which began operation in 1833. She taught her students music at the school.

Once during her time there, she was attending Mass at St. James Church in New York City. Suddenly there was a loud crash followed by screams caused a panic as the church's ceiling fell in on the sanctuary. People ran every which way for fear of further collapse.

Sister Euphemia's companion sister took refuge in the sacristy and lost consciousness. When she came to, she looked around for Sister Euphemia, whom she thought had followed her into the sacristy.

The sister walked back into the church and saw Sister Euphemia sitting quietly in her pew. The new sister was pale but composed. Sister Euphemia hadn't moved at all during the incident.[7]

Though now in her twenties, Sister Euphemia held onto her youthful zeal for her vocation of service to others. While that gave her the energy to work for God, her decorum was not always what was expected of a Sister of Charity. For instance, there were times she was caught running through the school at times to get from place to place more quickly.[8]

Though her spirit remained energetic, Sister Euphemia's body began to wear down under the weight of the work she took upon herself.

> Only a child in years, of a delicate constitution, and unaccustomed to labor, she experienced great fatigue, and no wonder, for after having spent long, trying hours in a classroom that held few conveniences and fewer comforts, she had to do her share of the general housework. Sometimes, overcome by weariness, she would fall asleep during night prayers.[9]

Sister Euphemia was recalled to Emmitsburg in 1841 and given the duty as the organist for the sisters. Sister Williamanna Hickey, a companion of Sister Euphemia's in New York, wrote, "I hope Sister Euphemia will do justice to the organ. I am quite proud of her office and that my old child is already so useful. I hope this weighty burden will not deprive her of her charity and love for 'Auld lang syne.'"[10]

Sister Euphemia's health did not improve as expected and so she was sent back to New York in 1842 for treatment at Mount Saint Vincent's Hospital, which later became Mount Hope. While there, she maintained a positive outlook about her treatment and others around her. Her compassion toward others in pain deepened as she dealt with her own pains. One student of

Sister Euphemia wrote of her disposition:

> Her daily life was like a tranquilizing melody bringing
> peace and solace to all who came within the sphere of her
> influence. To the remarkable amenity of her temper was
> added a rare combination of apparently opposite qualities:
> deep and lasting affection, that never conflicted with the
> fulfillment of sterner duties; a sensitive and refined nature
> that never yielded to repugnance or disgust where there
> was question of ministering to a physical or moral evil; a
> sweet condescension unbiased by human respect;
> cheerfulness without levity; gravity without moroseness
> or stiffness; perfect self-possession in presence of
> unforeseen and trying circumstances without the slightest
> shadow of self-assertion; a gracious dignity untainted by
> pride in worldliness. All these excellent qualifications
> united in making Sister Euphemia a peerless woman and a
> shining light among the Daughters of Charity.[11]

Sister Euphemia eventually recovered her health and was assigned as the Sister Servant at St. Peter's School in Baltimore in
1850. And so, Sister Euphemia returned to the city where her
family lived and where she had first made her decision to become a Sister of Charity.

The four Daughters of Charity who were already assigned to
St. Peter's School had spent a lot of time preparing the new Sister Servant's room and cleaning the house. Though not luxurious,
the sisters did what they could to make a comfortable home for
their new sister.

When Sister Euphemia arrived at the house, she smiled ap-
provingly at all of the work done on her behalf. The sisters
showed Sister Euphemia her new room with a little amount of
pride at what they had been able to accomplish.

One of the sisters had been recovering from illness, a fact that
did not escape Sister Euphemia's notice. "Sister, dear, we are

James Rada, Jr.

going to make a little exchange," Sister Euphemia said. "You will occupy the room prepared for me while I take your bed in the dormitory."[12]

Sister Euphemia remained at the school before being reassigned to St. Mary's Asylum, which was also in Baltimore. The asylum was in actuality an orphanage for girls, and it tested Sister Euphemia's compassion to the utmost.

In one instance a mother burned to death in a fire when the lamp in her home exploded. However, as her last act of life and love, she managed to shove her infant away from her. The action saved the child's life but left the baby's hand badly burned.

When Sister Euphemia saw the baby, she decided that she would care for the young girl. Sister Euphemia said that she was unwilling for her fellow sisters to be burdened more or to lose sleep because of the frequent cries of the child. So she kept the baby in a crib near her own bed, and she took care of the baby.

The child thrived under Sister Euphemia's attention, but the little girl's hand was forever disfigured. While some believed an operation might offer some help for the hand, Sister Euphemia would not consent because she thought the child would be put through too much pain without any benefit.

As the baby grew older, she spoke her first word, "Phemie." During the day, the baby was in the community room, and as Sister Euphemia would pass near in her duties, she would call out, "Phemie!"

Sister Euphemia would always stop and say, "Yes, Emma."

The baby eventually began crawling and walking and move through the house. Finally, the baby's grandfather located the child and took her to live with him in Chicago.[13]

In 1855, Sister Euphemia returned to Emmitsburg to serve as Mother Regina Smith's assistant. Even in her more-administrative role, she continued to give her heart to the people around her.

One elderly sister had grown so frail and her vision so poor that her duties had become limited. However, the older woman

88

would regularly come to Sister Euphemia's office for yarn to knit stockings for the other sisters.

"Thank God, dear, I can still knit for the community," the elderly sister would say.

When the woman completed a set of stockings, she would bring them to Sister Euphemia who accepted them with gratitude and thanks although the stockings would be full of holes from dropped stitches that the elderly sister couldn't see because of her poor eyesight. Sister Euphemia would then unravel the socks and ball the yarn back up for the next time the sister requested it.[14]

However, she was also known to be firm when needed and a supportive mentor and good leader of her fellow sisters. Such skills would be required as Mother Ann Simeon's representative in the Southern States.

Father Burlando once said of Sister Euphemia, "She is worth her weight in gold, and she is not very light!"[15]

The same day Sister Euphemia was named as Mother Ann Simeon's representative in the Confederate States of America, the Council of St. Joseph's also named one sister to serve in the military hospital in St. Louis and two sisters to work in Richmond, demonstrating the impartiality of the mission the Daughters of Charity were serving.[16]

On November 3, 1861, Sister Euphemia left Emmitsburg to take charge of the Southern missions accompanied by eight other sisters. The trip south began with a stagecoach ride to Washington and then a boat trip down the Chesapeake Bay on the steamer *Adelaide*.

Norfolk was still floating the Confederate flag. The Adelaide ran up to the danger line and a shot came crashing through her bow. A Confederate boat steamed out and took the passengers and all non-contraband goods; then it put back to shore.[17]

James Rada, Jr.

After a couple days in Norfolk visiting with other Daughters of Charity who were serving in St. Mary's Asylum and the naval hospital in Portsmouth, the group journeyed on to Richmond.

The good work of the sisters was suddenly jeopardized in December 1861 as the ease with which the sisters moved across the border between North and South was noticed by other people who hadn't taken a neutral position in the war.

On December 17, Francis Patrick Kenrick, Archbishop of Baltimore, wrote to Father Burlando that Daughters of Charity had caused some alarm in military circles. Union Major General John Adams Dix had leveled a charge "that ladies dressed in the costume of Sisters of Charity furnished by the convent at Emmitsburg, have passed the lines into Virginia, for the purpose of keeping up communication with the Confederate States."[18]

Archbishop Kenrick had explained to Dix "that the Sisters were stationed at Richmond and Norfolk for many years and they have extended their services to the sick and wounded, and from time to time, they visited the parent institution which supplied them with the dress of their order; and regulated their domestic relations. I informed him that these journeys have ceased, a Sister being permanently in charge of the rest. I also stated that their journeys were open and with formal passports from the Government at Washington, and wholly unconnected with politics, and not intended in any way to aid rebellion."[19]

The Council of St. Joseph's also wrote General Dix to clarify "that at no time, under no circumstances, directly or indirectly, have any Sisters belonging to said Community gone to Virginia or any other state for political purposes, or carried documents or messages having political tendencies. The only object for which the Sisters were sent to Virginia was to nurse the sick and wounded soldiers."[20]

They explained that a sister had been appointed to represent Mother Ann Simeon in the South so that there should be no further problems caused by sisters traveling across the border. However, they also pointed out that just because the sisters helped in the South did not mean they were disloyal to the Union. They helped just as much in the North with the sick and wounded.

In a word: the Sisters have responded to every call without distinction of creed or politics, and are ready at the moment to give their services if asked by the proper authority ... they are willing to suspend their schools and diminish their number in hospitals and orphan asylums for the purpose of nursing the sick and the wounded. Of about eight hundred Sisters of Charity, there is not one but would readily obey the first summons for the same work of charity.[21]

The council replied that the problem may have been a woman impersonating one of the sisters since it had happened before.

This may be possible as, about the twenty-fifth of last October, two individuals alleging to be from the South, dressed like Sisters, were seen in Baltimore, feigning to be nieces of the Honorable E. Everett, both of whom are members of our Community. The Sisters were much mortified and felt indignant at the imposition. We take the liberty to remark that the duty of the Sisters of Charity is to strive to save their souls by the exercise of charity towards their fellow-creatures, the poor and suffering of every nation, independent of creed or politics.[22]

With this response, the sisters were no longer able to travel between the North and the South without a permit. However, the move that the Council of St. Joseph's had taken with Sister Euphemia allowed their work to continue in the South. She had arrived at St. Simeon's School in New Orleans. Sister Mathilde Duvernay wrote:

I remember it well. We had a dear little organ, small but with a soft, melodious tone. We asked Sister Assistant to exercise her old profession and be organist for the occasion and she consented. Wasn't it condescending! We had practiced the Mass well so as to have it very nice. It was Andre's Mass. Father [Hayden] Hayden, the Visitor,[23] was the celebrant.[24]

Another sister wrote years later of what Sister Euphemia's visit meant to her:

The only ray of consolation during this trying period, dear Mother, was your short visit to us. It served to delight and cheer us for many a long month after and nerved us to go through the terrible times that followed.[25]

Two days after Christmas, the Council of St. Joseph's named four more sisters to serve in the military hospital in St. Louis.

In Alabama, Sister Gabriella Rigney who ran City Hospital in Mobile wrote Father Burlando after the war, saying:

During the first year of the war; the Confederate Governor asked for Sisters to take charge of their sick and wounded. About the second year of the war, we had to take in our Hospital the Confederate sick besides the city patients and occasionally Federal Prisoners were sent to us.[26]

When the holidays ended, Sister Euphemia returned to Richmond. Had she stayed in New Orleans much longer, she would have been cut off from the Southern missions she had been sent to serve. New Orleans fell to the Union Army on April 23, 1862.

CHAPTER 8
1862

"The Sisters of Charity were able to lessen the cares and labors of the physicians and surgeons in any hospital they might be placed in. "

First Surgeon
Satterlee Hospital

Although the war had split the country and the Daughters of Charity's efforts were being spent caring for wounded soldiers both in the North and the South, the sisters still sought to continue their other missions of educating children, mothering the orphaned and caring for the sick. While many of the sisters were involved in war work east of the Mississippi River, others worked in the west at other duties.

In January 1862, Sister Francis McGinnis wrote to Father Burlando about the sisters in San Francisco, California, under Sister Scholastica Logsdon.

It has been raining for the last six weeks; all the country is flooded and hundreds and thousands of poor people are flocking to San Francisco. We have offered our services to take care of the children, and we are crowded ... The poor farmers have lost every thing in the world; all the grain in the country is washed away. Flour is going up very high. . . . We have lost nothing from our farm. ... All the neighbors round our place lost their cows, hones, chickens, etc. [1]

* * *

93

James Rada, Jr.

The Daughters of Charity operated St. Joseph's Seminary in San Francisco. It was founded in 1860 even as it became apparent that there would be a war between the states. At the end of 1860, Sister Scholastica had written Father Burlando about what the seminary would be.

The best plan…is to purchase a house for the Sick and take the one we use now for them for the school. We can buy a very pretty property of seven acres newly planted in choice fruit trees and grape vines with a new brick house sufficiently large for our present wants for the sick … for between six and seven thousand dollars by paying three thousand in hand when the deed is delivered. … The house is about the same distance from our house as the deaf and dumb institution is from St. Joseph's. … We can have private rooms for the patents which will aid us in time for the support of the Seminary.[2]

At times, staffing in the west or in schools and orphanages run by the Daughters of Charity suffered as the need for nurses grew in the east, but the sisters always moved forward in their work.

On January 9, 1862, five sisters left Richmond for Manassas. Dr. Thomas Williams, the medical director of the Army of the Potomac, had requested their help. When they arrived in Manassas, Sister Angela Heath wrote:

We were five in number and found on taking possession, 500 patients, sick and wounded of both armies. Mortality was very great, as the poor sick had been very much neglected. The wards were in the most deplorable condition, and strongly resisted all efforts of the broom to which they had long been strangers, and the aid of a shovel was found necessary. At best, they were but poor protection

94

against the inclemency of the season, and being scattered, we were often obliged to go through snow over a foot deep, to wait on the sick.[3]

Sister Euphemia also traveled from Richmond to see what the sisters were doing among the wounded there. She brought two sisters with her to help the Daughters of Charity already working in Manassas. As Sister Euphemia attempted to leave the rail car at the Manassas station, she was stopped by a Confederate sentry who had never seen a Daughter of Charity before and didn't know what to make of their religious attire.

"Don't you know us?" Sister Euphemia asked. "We are Sisters of Charity. Some of our sisters are taking care of your men."

The sentry was saved from having to decide what to do with the arrival of two medical directors. One of the men had been a student at Charity Hospital and the other at the Baltimore Infirmary. Both of them were well acquainted with the Daughters of Charity even if they didn't know Sister Euphemia. They dressed down the sentry for holding up a sister whose help was needed among the wounded.

Rather than take offense at the sentry's questioning, Sister Euphemia said, "He was only doing his duty."[4]

The sisters' quarters in Manassas consisted of one room, which was used for a chapel, dormitory, and refectory. Sister Angela wrote, "The kitchen to which, what was called the refectory, was attached, was a quarter of a mile away from the Sisters' room and often it was found more prudent to be satisfied with two meals a day than to trudge through the snow and sleet for the third."[5] These meals, at best, were not very inviting because the culinary department was under the care of slaves who had no concern about cleanliness.

Sister Euphemia brought tea with her for the sisters. It was a luxury for anyone to have real tea at the time and greatly appreciated.[6] She stayed only a few days before she needed to return to Richmond, but the Daughters of Charity were at Manassas for two months.

When the Daughters of Charity were forced to leave for a new assignment in March, they still had 500 patients under their care. The Confederacy was forced to retreat from the area, and the sisters had six hours to move out. "[T]hey had scarcely left their posts when the whole camp was one mass of flames and the bodies of those who died that day were consumed."[7]

Three sisters moved with the army to the military hospital in Gordonsville, Virginia. The Exchange Hotel, which had been built two years earlier to serve as a railroad hotel for the Virginia Central Railway, had been converted to the Gordonsville Receiving and Distributing Hospital along with some of the other buildings in the town. The three-story Georgian-style hotel was the primary hotel, though, and it admitted 23,000 wounded and injured soldiers during its first year as a hospital.[8]

When the Daughters of Charity arrived in Gordonsville, they had 200 patients suffering from pneumonia or typhus to care for. The sisters had no beds on which to sleep for the first week; they used their habits and a shawl lent to them by one of the doctors for bed coverings. A tree trunk served as their table, and they drank from the rusty cups and ate off the plates in everyday use.[9] The sisters had a small room which served all purposes for all of them.

The Daughters of Charity cared for the sick and wounded in Gordonsville for six weeks. Sister Euphemia visited them there to view their work and working conditions.

While visiting these Camps, Sister Euphemia saw that the Sisters' opportunities for doing good were greatly hampered; that the Sister often had to sleep on the ground with only a little straw for a bed; and finally, that they were very much exposed; so she determined to send them either to some stationary hospitals or back to their respective missions.[10]

* * *

However, the good sister was stopped by a question from Father Aegidius Smulders, the Redemptorist army chaplain. He asked, "And who will be responsible for the souls that might have been saved?"

He claimed that hundreds of souls would have been lost without the agency of the Sisters, for they had instructed these poor fellows, who were so ignorant in matters of faith that in the exercise of his sacred ministry, he would have but little success without their aid. Won by his representation, Sister Euphemia yielded to the urgent need and concluded that our Sisters must remain at the front to continue the good work wherein the Community was reaping so rich a harvest in the salvation of souls.[11]

The sisters found that the soldiers knew little about Christianity. When one of the sisters was explaining the Passion of Our Divine Savior to them, a soldier voicing his surprise and sympathy exclaimed: "Poor fellow! I guess if we had been there, those Jews that nailed Him to the cross would have caught something!"[12]

By late April, Sister Euphemia wanted to visit the sisters in New Orleans, which was under control of the Union Army, but when she applied for a travel pass, she was told to wait for a day or two.

She returned to Richmond where there was always work for her to do caring for the wounded soldiers. On May 2, she sent three sisters to the military hospital at Danville, Virginia. The 400 patients there were better cared for than those on Manassas or Gordonsville, but the sisters were living in worse conditions. Rats carried off their shoes, stockings and even nibbled on their fingers and toes.[13]

A Northern steward and a Southern surgeon became involved in a personal dispute which ended by one challenging the other to meet him in a retired spot near the battlefield. Both withdrew towards an old shed and at the same time continued to threaten each other in loud angry tones. No one interfered with them and the duel would have taken place had not one of the Sisters followed them. She spoke to them firmly and reproachfully, took their pistols away from them, and the affair ended by their separating like docile children, each retiring to his post. It was on valiant women this stern type that Mother Ann Simeon could count to carry on the work of God.[14]

Back in the north, Father Burlando sought permission to open a new hospital in Baltimore staffed by the Daughters of Charity to expand health care for the poor. He wrote to Archbishop Kenrick about his idea and even suggested calling the hospital Carroll Hospital or any name the archbishop might want.[15] The new hospital became St. Agnes Hospital after the wife of the major donor who purchased the property and erected the facility.

Father Burlando followed up that letter with one to the medical faculty of the Baltimore Infirmary.

Favorable circumstances induce the Sisters of Charity to open a hospital for the poor in Baltimore; in consequence of this the central Council of the Sisters has decided to withdraw Sisters from the Baltimore Infirmary and place them in the institution about to commence. . . . The long uninterrupted harmonious connection between the Sisters and the Baltimore Infirmary cause the Superiors of the Sisters to regret the step.[16]

So many things needed to be done and even more needed his attention at this time. He was like the Commander-in-Chief. While he might be fighting a war,—in Father Burlando's case, it wasn't the War Between the States; he was fighting man's inhumanity against man--he also had other duties to attend to. The sister's needed to be sent where their nursing skills were needed, but there were still children in the Daughter of Charity orphanages, children who needed to be taught, civilians who needed medical attention, people everywhere who needed to hear the Gospel of Jesus Christ and the poor who needed help getting back on their feet. If the war had ended the next day, Father Burlando still would have been a very busy man.

On May 25, 1862, Union Surgeon General William H. Hammond asked for twenty-five sisters to nurse the sick and wounded soldiers at West Philadelphia Hospital, which would soon become known as Satterlee General Hospital, named after Dr. Walter Satterlee of Philadelphia. This hospital would become the largest Union hospital during the war. It was located between Spruce and Pine streets and 40th to 44th streets.[17]

The Daughter of Charity placed in charge of this huge hospital was Sister Mary Gonzaga Grace. She was fifty years old and serving at the Saint Joseph's Orphan Asylum in Philadelphia when asked to coordinate the nursing care at Satterlee. Besides patient care, the sisters also oversaw the kitchen and storeroom at the hospital.[18]

Sister Mary Gonzaga Grace had been born Mary Agnes Grace in 1812 in Baltimore and baptized in Saint Patrick's Church there. She left Baltimore in December 1823 to attend Saint Joseph's Academy in Emmitsburg. She spent four years there and was an excellent student. It was also at the academy where she began considering devoting her life to God.

She entered the Sisters of Charity on March 11, 1827, and a year later she went on her first mission to help two other sisters open a free school and asylum in Harrisburg, Pennsylvania.

Once the school was firmly established, the Council of St. Joseph's sent Sister Mary Gonzaga east to Philadelphia in May 1830 to Saint Joseph's Orphan's Asylum, which was connected to the Holy Trinity Church. The orphanage was moved to a new location in 1836 and Sister Mary Gonzaga, three other sisters and fifty-one children went with it.

It was a turbulent time for Catholics in the city, but the sisters continued their mission undeterred. "Here she went on with her good work, placid and calm in the midst of the worrying turbulence of anti-Catholic bitterness and persecution, which at times threatened the lives of innocent women and children,"[19] wrote George Barton in *Angels of the Battlefield.*

Sister Mary Gonzaga was sent to Donaldsonville, Louisiana, in 1844 to serve as an assistant in the newly established Novitiate, which formed with postulants from the South as Sisters of Charity. The following year she was transferred to New Orleans, only to return to Saint Joseph's Asylum in March 1851.

In 1855, she spent a year at the Mother House in France in an administrative capacity and then returned to the Central House in Emmitsburg to serve as Procuratrix or housekeeper for the community.

In January 1857, she returned to Saint Joseph's Asylum in Philadelphia for the third time and remained in charge there until assuming responsibilities at Satterlee, where her gift for administration would be honed to a sharp edge.

Workmen were still constructing the buildings of the hospital when Sister Mary Gonzaga and twenty-one Daughters of Charity arrived on June 9 at 10 a.m.[20] The hospital was so large that the sisters couldn't find the entrance at first.[21]

> The workmen looked at us in amazement, thinking
> perhaps that we belonged to the Flying Artillery [because
> of our large white cornettes]; after stepping over bricks,
> mortar, pipes &-e [& etc.]we were ushered in to an
> immense ward while a good Irishman went in search of
> the Surgeon in charge; he [Dr. Hayes] and his staff
> welcomed us, showed us our quarters and desired us to
> order dinner to [be] sent ourselves; he then showed us
> through the Hospital, of which 8 wards only were
> finished, their number when completed was 33, each
> capable of accommodating comfortably 75 patients each

having a table & chair... the Hospital grounds covered a space of fifteen acres, giving our sick ample space to move about and recreate themselves.[22]

Within a month, the hospital would have 3,000 beds in thirty-three wards. More than half of those beds would be filled in another month.

The sisters' first meal at Satterlee Hospital showed the incompleteness of the preparations to receive them. The sisters were served tea in thick pitchers and meat and potatoes in basins. They were given no forks or knives. When they asked the cook for utensils, he told them that there were only four and they were for the officers. However, since the officers wouldn't eat until later, he allowed the sisters to use them in turns.[23]

Their accommodations at the hospital were no better. The sisters had one small room that was around seven feet square that served as their chapel. "When we had Mass, there was only room for a few Sisters to remain inside, and at the time for Holy Communion they were obliged to come out, in order that they outside might have their turn to receive,"[24] wrote Sister Mary Gonzaga.

Another room was slightly larger since it had to house all of the sisters for their sleeping.

When smallpox broke out at Satterlee, the patients were segregated in a hospital facility miles away from the city. Sister Mary Gonzaga wrote that the men were distressed at being taken from the care of the sisters. "It was heart-rending when the ambulance came to hear the poor fellows begging to be left, even if they had to be entirely alone, provided the Sisters would be near them to have the Sacraments administered in the hour of danger," Sister Mary Gonzaga wrote.[25]

The reason given for not allowing the sisters to venture out to the smallpox hospital was because it was so far away and the sisters were needed at Satterlee. Sister Mary Gonzaga noted:

We offered our services several times to attend these poor sick, but were told the Government had ordered them away to prevent the contagion spreading. At last our Surgeon in charge obtained permission to keep the small pox patients in the camp some distance from the Hospital, the Tents were made very comfortable with good large stoves to heat them and flies (double covers) over the tops; the next thing was to have a Sister in readiness in case their services should be required; every one was generous enough to offer her service, but I thought it most prudent to accept one who had had the disease."[26]

Once they heard that a sister had been assigned to help them, the soldiers said, "Well, if I get the small pox now, I don't care because our sister will take care of me."[27]

In mid-June, Surgeon General Hammond asked the Council of St. Joseph's for 100 sisters to go to "The White House" on the Pamunkey River in Virginia, "that graceful green slope on the Virginia side of the Potomac opposite Washington, where the wounded waited for hospital boats that would carry them north."[28]

General George McClellan had chosen White House Landing to serve as his primary supply base for his Army of the Potomac during its operations against Richmond in 1862. It served as such from the third week of May until June 29, 1862. Mary Custis Lee (Mrs. Robert E. Lee) had taken refuge here until May, departing just before the Union troops assumed its control. General McClellan guaranteed her safe passage to Richmond. With Mrs. Lee's departure, the place became an immense hospital as the campaign evolved.

Hammond's telegram arrived at St. Joseph's and was taken to Father Burlando. He called the council together that same night. It was decided to have sisters from various missions meet in Baltimore. Father Burlando traveled from Emmitsburg to Baltimore with some of the sisters to join the group gathering there.

From Baltimore, sixty Daughters of Charity traveled by ship down the Chesapeake Bay and then up the Potomac River, a circuitous route to be sure. Major Robert Langdon Eastman was among the soldiers who welcomed the sisters' arrival at White House Landing.

News came that the old transport was bringing sisters to nurse the sick and wounded, and when the whistle sounded off the wharf hundreds rushed to the shore lining the banks, as a band of gentle, devoted women stepped ashore, their white bonnets waving like the wings of pigeons, a lane-way opened through the crowd and as they marched to the ambulances, hats flew off and words of welcome and blessing filled the air; and as they drove to various camp hospitals an enormous cheer went up that brought the enemy to alert watchfulness, thinking, as they said afterward, that we had received news of a great victory, or that some new campaign movement was begun.[29]

The number of wounded at White House Landing had been growing because many of the hospital ships had already left Virginia and headed north. At this time, the U.S. Sanitary Commission controlled the hospital ships, and one of the complaints about their administration of the ships was that they sailed even if the ships weren't completely filled and many of the patients weren't severely wounded or ill. This meant that more serious cases were left in the makeshift hospitals at White House Landing.[30]

Major Eastman recalled when the sisters arrived:

Words of welcome and blessing filled the air, and as they drove to the various hospitals an enormous cheer went up that brought the enemy to alert watchfulness, thinking, as they said afterward, that we had received news of a great victory, or that some new campaign movement had begun.[31]

Despite the enthusiasm to their arrival, Father Burlando and the sisters found that no accommodations had been made for them. He spent the next day unsuccessfully trying to make arrangements for the sisters. Discouraged, he was ready to return home when he met Col. Butler, the commander of the camp, whom he told of his decision to remove the sisters from the area.

He asked if there was any possibility of retaining them. I answered, yes, if a proper place could be found for them. He gave me a pass to examine the White House. I found it suitable, if some additional accommodations could be provided. This I represented to the Colonel and it took yesterday and Sunday to come to a conclusion. Last evening the answer came from General McClellan that the sisters could occupy the White House.[32]

Though the shaded grounds and the large house would have made a good hospital, General McClellan wanted to protect what he considered a landmark. So he posted guards around the property to keep soldiers off of it.[33]

Eighty sisters stayed in White House Landing and, in many respects, they were better accommodated than the officers at White House Landing.[34]

While waiting for assignments, the Daughters of Charity cared for 1,150 soldiers brought there from various battlefields. They fed them, washed them and changed their bandages.

The day after Father Burlando found the sisters accommodations, Dr. Dunster arrived with Sister Camilla O'Keefe and thirty more sisters. Some sisters were assigned to help on the steamboats *Vanderbilt* and *Commodore* while others would remain at White House Landing to help. At first, the doctors on the transports did not welcome the sisters' help, but that attitude changed in a short time.[35]

Among the sisters working on the ships, Sister Euphrasia Mattingly wrote about patients being stacked on the floor of all of the decks so that the ships became so overloaded that it was "more like sinking than sailing." She described being below decks as having no air and being lit by candles and lamps day and night.[36]

> When men, sisters, provisions, horses, etc. were all on
> board, we were more like sinking than sailing…Here mis-
> ery was in her fullness and her victims testified to her
> power by the thousand-toned moans of bitter
> waves.…Here our sisters shared with their poor patients
> every horror except that of feeling their bodily pains.
> They were in the lower cabins; the ceiling low, and light-
> ed all day by hanging lamps or candles; the men dying on
> the floor with only space to stand or kneel between
> them.[37]

Once the sisters settled into the White House and their new duties, Father Burlando left on the *Vanderbilt* and headed for Norfolk and Portsmouth. He wrote:

> I trust I shall not have so much to suffer there as in this
> place. But, perhaps God wished to try us that we might be
> convinced that it is He Who is to furnish the Sisters with
> the opportunity of doing good.[38]

Despite McClellan's respect for Lee, it didn't stop their two armies from battling from June 25 to July 1 in the Seven Days Battle. The Union forces were forced to withdraw to Harrison's Landing on the James River.

> Here was a scene of confusion baffling description and of
> additional suffering to the sick. The poor wounded and

dying soldiers had to be conveyed to the transport ships; when men, Sisters, horses, and provisions were on board, the vessels seemed ready to sink. The Sisters had to attend the sick, but how was it possible to relieve their pressing wants? Here misery reigned supreme and victims testified to its tyranny by their bitter moans and groans." Sisters were asked to accompany to their places of safety. "Our Sisters shared every horror with their poor patients save their bodily pains. They were in the lower cabins which were lighted all day by hanging lamps and candles; the ceiling was very low; the space between the men's beds on the floor was so narrow that it allowed room only for one to stand or kneel. The Sister in charge of the lower ward (Sister Henrietta Casey) was so persevering in her zealous attentions that even the doctor declared that he did not see how human nature could endure such a strain. But her charity was to her energy what the oil of her lamp was to her vision. Self was forgotten save as an hourly oblation to God's glory and her neighbor's salvation. She seemed perfectly unconscious that she was being observed by any one; it was enough for her that God was there, and though she was then about forty years' vocation such had been her sole aim throughout her life.[39]

The sisters in Richmond also experienced the Seven Days Battle. Sister Juliana Chatard noted that the fighting was constant from 2 a.m. each day until 10 p.m. at night:

All kinds of misery lay outstretched before us. A terrible engagement commencing near the City, this hospital being more convenient was made the field hospital, where all the wounded were first brought, their wounds examined and dressed, then sent to other hospitals to make room for others. The Battle lasted 7 days, commencing about 2:00 a.m. and continuing to 10 p.m. each day. The bombs were bursting and reddening the heavens while the Reserve Corps ranged about three hundred yards from our door. While these days lasted, our poor Sisters in the City Hospitals were shaken by the cannonading and the heavy rolling of the ambulances filling the streets bringing in the wounded and dying men. The entire city trembled as if from an earthquake of a few short hours between 10 and 2:00 o'clock. Memory is surfeited over these days; hearts overflowing with anguish at the bare remembrance of them.[40]

Nine thousand sick and wounded soldiers needed hospital beds in Richmond during and after the fighting. One Confederate surgeon wrote to his wife:

The most saddening sight was the wounded at the hospitals, which were in various places on the battlefield. Not only are the houses full, but even the yards are covered with them. There are so many that most of them are much neglected. The people of Richmond are hauling them away as fast as possible. At one place I saw the Yankee wounded and their own surgeons attending them. There are no crops or fences anywhere, and I saw nothing which had escaped the Yankees except one little Guinea fowl.[41]

Realizing that a lot of fighting would happen in the region around Richmond, the Confederate government had added to the number of beds in the city. Pavilions at the west end of Cary Street at the edge of the city were built to hold 4,000 to 5,000 patients and called Winder Hospital. The 98 buildings had good water sources with both wells and springs, a library, information house, cook-houses, bakeries, food-processing facilities, employee barracks, treatment and medical buildings, warehouses, 125 acres of farmland used for growing supplies, recreational facilities, and bathhouses. It even had regular transportation service to down-

James Rada, Jr.

town Richmond and operated own river and canal boats.

The medical service took over the barracks on Chimborazo Hill in October 1861 to create an even larger hospital facility. The Chimborazo Hospital had 120 building and a medical staff of forty-five. The hospital had its own ice house, soup house, bakery, and soap factory. Like Winder, Chimborazo Hospital operated its own farms with beef and goat herds to have enough food to feed the thousands of people at the hospital.

The Confederate officers even took steps to protect the asset they knew they had with the Daughters of Charity. The officers believed that Union soldiers were under orders to capture the Catholic sisters if they could in an attempt to undermine the Confederate medical system. The sisters were warned of this so that they could take precautions.[42]

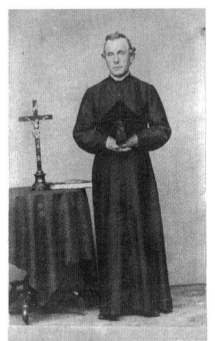

Father Peter McCrane served at Satterlee Hospital. Courtesy of Philadelphia Archdiocean Historical Research Center.

108

CHAPTER 9
The Voice of Experience

"Within the sound of my voice, and within this courtroom, is one who upon the bloody field of Gettysburg I saw bending over the dying and the dead – binding up with her own hands the prostrate soldier's wounds, or commending, with her earnest prayers, his departing spirit to the mercy of his God."

William P. Preston
Attorney

On June 4, 1862, about 400 soldiers had arrived at the U.S. Military Hospital in Frederick, Maryland. The Union Army at the order of Brigadier General Nathaniel Banks had created the military hospital on the outskirts of Frederick the prior August. It was located in stone barracks that had once housed George Washington's colonial army during the Revolutionary War and, later in the Revolutionary War, it was a prison for soldiers.

Most of the soldiers suffered from typhoid and dysentery, and the medical authorities were not prepared to receive them. The doctors requested the help of the Daughters of Charity in caring for the sick and wounded soldiers. They telegraphed a message to the Central House in Emmitsburg, twenty-four miles to the north, asking for ten sisters to help in Frederick. However, the demand for the Daughters of Charity's services had stretched their resources thin. Only three sisters from Emmitsburg were available to send, but the Council of Saint Joseph's managed to arrange for seven additional sisters to travel to Frederick from

James Rada, Jr.

Baltimore. Upon their arrival in Frederick, one sister wrote:

> Meanwhile, the Chief Surgeon called to welcome us and
> hoped that we would be comfortable in our military quar-
> ters. He also said that we were to call upon the steward
> for whatever we wanted but, thank God, we had enough
> when we saw the condition of the poor wounded soldiers
> who were without food and nourishment enough, and
> even that was ill prepared. The medicines were plentiful,
> but badly administered by the male and female nurses
> who did not seem to attach much importance to the time
> or manner of giving them.[1]

Because the hospital was so overcrowded, many of the soldiers who arrived on June 4 lay in the hospital yard for almost a
day while Sisters Matilda Coskery, Mary Alice Thomas, and Do-
nata Bell tried to provide some relief and find beds for them.
Finally, Sister Matilda managed to find some wine. She watered
it down to increase the volume and was able to provide the suffering soldiers with a refreshing drink without overwhelming
their ill systems.[2]

"A nurse may suppose that thirst must be allayed whenever it
is great & then allow free drinks unmindful of quantity or quality
– This is sometimes of a very serious moment, as it either
overloads the weak stomach, or causes it to be vomited, much to
the inconvenience or injury of the patient," Sister Matilda wrote
in *Advices Concerning the Sick.*[3]

The stream of incoming patients didn't let up and the chief
surgeon soon had to take over a few of the larger public buildings
in the city to use for hospitals.[4] The Daughters of Charity also
found eight more sisters to send to the city to help in the additional buildings.

The sisters' accommodations were no better than the soldiers.
They had a small room in the old Hessian barracks. The ten beds
were jammed together with an old table and a couple of chairs

that threatened to collapse if someone sat in them.

The sisters ate soldiers' rations served to them on broken plates with rusty utensils. The patients told the sisters, "There is no necessity for the doctors to order us the tincture of iron three times a day; don't you think we get nearly enough of it off our table service?"[5]

Because the patients also complained about the quality of the food they were served, the Council of St. Joseph's sent a sister to supervise the kitchen at the request of the Chief Surgeon.[6] "Nothing should be thought small in the mind of the Nurse, where the benefit or injury of her patient is in question," Sister Matilda wrote.[7]

Not only did she believe this, but she had also learned it over her many years of working with the sick and afflicted.

Sister Matilda Coskery was born Anastasia Coskery on November 21, 1799, near Taneytown, Maryland. She was the second of eight children that Jacoba and John Coskery would have.

It's not known why Coskery felt drawn to a religious life. Most likely, it was a gradual process affected in part by relatives who had entered the religious life and others who attended St. Joseph's Free School and Academy.

Coskery sought to become a Sister of Charity in 1828 and Reverend Nicholas Zocchi, pastor of the St. Joseph Catholic Church in Taneytown recommended her. The Sisters of Charity accepted her application on July 7. She was admitted to the seminary and given the name of Sister Matilda on August 15, 1829.

Her first mission was to Mount St. Mary's College and Seminary in Emmitsburg to nurse in the infirmary there and in serving that mission, she discovered a life calling to heal the sick and wounded.[8] Sister Matilda eventually became the Infirmarian-Nurse at Mount St. Mary's College where her duties included "that she gave nothing to the sick which could cause them harm; that she did not tell them anything which could sadden them, or anything which is said at the House; that she gave nothing which was served at the sisters' meals."[9]

In 1833, she was sent to help the insane at the Maryland Hospital, a public city hospital in Baltimore. The Sisters of Charity had taken over the administration of the hospital under the supervision of the Maryland General Assembly. The doctors at the hospital treated diseases like epilepsy, gangrene, and syphilis.

The year after Sister Matilda arrived, the mission of the hospital changed. No longer could they admit patients with contagious diseases. Instead, they began to treat mental illnesses. Besides prescription medications, the sisters worked with herbal remedies and opium tinctures to treat mental illness. They also took a holistic approach to treatment, making sure patients exercised, engaging them in conversation and trying to amuse them.

Sister Matilda became the Sister Servant at the Richmond Medical College in Richmond, in 1838 and served there until 1840. The new hospital grew under her direction as did her own knowledge of patient care.

In 1840, the Sisters of Charity brought property on Harford Road in Baltimore to open their own hospital for the insane called St. Vincent's. Sister Matilda was recalled from Richmond to open the new hospital. Not only did she have experience opening a hospital, but she also had experience dealing with the insane. It was quickly apparent to anyone who brought their loved ones to the hospital. As word of the quality care that patients received spread, admissions increased, and the hospital needed to be expanded.

The sisters worked to practice ethical treatment of the patients, which meant minimizing the use of restraints that was common at the time. They practiced kindness rather than severity.

Dr. William Stokes, who worked with the Sisters of Charity at St. Vincent's wrote, "We have endeavored, by our united efforts, to establish in this State a model Asylum, in which the patients should enjoy the utmost freedom, consistent with their own welfare, and the safety of others."[10]

Following a fire at St. Vincent's, the Sisters of Charity purchased the Mount Hope College in Baltimore and turned it into a hospital, which they moved into in 1844. There, they continued to offer the high level of care to sick that had caused the reputation of St. Vincent's to grow so quickly. A doctor who visited Mount Hope from New York wrote of it:

> The Mount Hope hospital is but a short distance from Baltimore; it belongs to the "Sisters of Charity," and is wholly under their management. Dr. Stokes, of Baltimore, visits it daily. He was at the hospital when we called, and with one of the Sisters accompanied us through the entire establishment, which we found very neat and in good order. The number of insane was about sixty, three-fourths of whom were women.[11]

Sister Matilda left Mount Hope in 1847. She returned to Emmitsburg for a few months of rest and then was off to New York to help manage and expand St. Patrick's Asylum in Rochester. The Sisters of Charity had assumed the administration of the hospital in 1845. She continued there until 1849 when she was recalled to Emmitsburg. From there, Sister Matilda served a short time in Norfolk and then was called to Detroit, Michigan, in 1850 to aid the sisters in combating a cholera epidemic there.

She remained there for two years until she was called to the mission at the Baltimore Infirmary and then St. Peter's Asylum in Wilmington, Delaware.

Since leaving Mount Hope, Sister Matilda's health had been deteriorating; though she was able to recover somewhat once, she was given time to do so.

It is believed that she began her instructional book, *Advices Concerning the Sick*, sometime in the 1850s, though the manuscript is not dated.[12] In this short text, Sister Matilda distilled her experience of how to best care for patients in a holistic way. It was advice that would prove valuable during the Civil War, even as she and the other Daughters of Charity learned even more about providing care. In this instance, it would be caring would the wounded and maimed rather than the sick and insane.

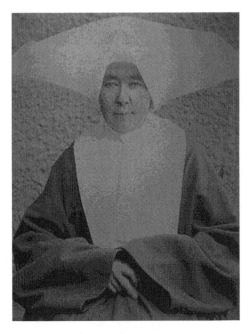

Sister Camilla O'Keefe had a variety of nursing experiences during the Civil War.
Courtesy of the Daughters of Charity.

CHAPTER 10
Losing a Daughter

*"News came that the old transport was bringing
Sisters to nurse the sick and wounded, and when
the whistle sounded off the wharf hundreds rushed
to the shore lining the banks, as a band of gentle,
devoted women stepped ashore, their white
bonnets waving like the wings of pigeons, a lane-
way opened through the crowd and as they
marched to the ambulances, hats flew off and
words of welcome and blessing filled the air; and
as they drove to the various camp hospitals an
enormous cheer went up that brought the enemy
to alert watchfulness, thinking, as they said
afterward, that we had received news of a great
victory, or that some new campaign movement
had begun."*

Major Robert Langdon Eastman
U.S. Army

On July 14, 1862, Father Burlando and twenty-six sisters
sailed from Baltimore for the hospital encampment at Point
Lookout and arrived the next day. Point Lookout was on the extreme Southern tip of Maryland. It was bounded by the Potomac
River on one side and the Chesapeake Bay on the other. The federal government built a lighthouse there in 1830, but the land
around it had been purchased by William Johnson who had plans
to develop a resort on the point until the war had refocused the
federal government's attention back to the point.[1]

James Rada, Jr.

When General George McClellan failed to capture Richmond earlier in the year, he had been left with wounded soldiers who needed care. The Union government had leased the land in June and built the Hammond Hospital, named for Surgeon General William Hammond.

Hammond Hospital consisted of twenty buildings erected on wooden pilings, so they were a few feet off the ground. This helped protect the hospital from flooding since the hospital was more than 500 feet long and it covered nearly all of Point Lookout. The hospital could accommodate up to 1,400 sick and wounded soldiers. The wings were arranged like sixteen spokes of a wheel radiating out from a central hub. Each wing was 175 feet long and 25 feet wide. The hospital offices lived in one wing, but the other fifteen were patient wards.[2]

The wards were connected by a covered circular walkway in the central hub. Four buildings also occupied the central hub area—the half-diet kitchen, library and reading room, chapel and baggage room. Each of these buildings was 77 feet long and 25 feet wide.[3]

The the other main feature of the hospital was the wharf that allowed wounded soldiers to be brought by ship directly to the hospital.[4] "As soon as a boat would land at the wharf, a horn was blown to let the Sisters know that they must go to their wards where they would assign the place of each [new patient], as to bed, etc., then give a little broth or wine, as was best to each."[5]

The Daughters of Charity had only been at Point Lookout for two weeks when Sister Consolata Conlon died from typhoid fever that she had contracted on the transport that brought the sisters to Point Lookout.[6] Sister Consolata was not the only Daughter of Charity who would die during the war, but she was the first and the one for whom the most-complete record exists.

Sister Consolata had only been a Daughter of Charity for a little over a year. However, in that year, she had served at Charity Hospital in New Orleans, Troy Hospital in New York and then on the field ambulances on the battlefield.

When her symptoms became alarming the Priest was sent for but as he was stationed twelve miles distant he could not get there in time; he arrived only to perform the burial service. Every mark of honor was rendered to this dear Sister by the doctors and officers; at her funeral they acted as pall-bearers. When the soldiers were buried their bodies were merely enveloped in a sheet because there was no lumber from which to make coffins, but they managed to obtain a white pine coffin for Sister. While the band played a funeral march, the procession including the authorities moved to the burial place. There on the banks of the Potomac the exhausted Sister of Charity was laid to rest but the prayers of Holy Church by the ministry of one of her faithful sons consecrated the spot. A martyr of charity had become the foundation of that new mission.[7]

On August 10, Dr. Bache of the military medical staff in New Orleans called on Sister Regina to send Sisters to the Marine Hospital to care for the sick soldiers arriving there. He had learned that 1,600 troops had left the Mississippi swamp where they had been encamped and would overwhelm the staff at the Marine Hospital, which had been converted to a Confederate military hospital until the Union had taken New Orleans in April. The wounded from the military hospital had been sent to Charity Hospital where they would be safe in the care of the Daughters of Charity.

The Union turned the Confederate military hospital into a Union one. Sister Regina was told to send three sisters to the hospital where 1,600 sick soldiers were expected from the Mississippi Swamp.

Sisters have been asked for, at least to superintend. These poor creatures [the soldiers] are generally protestants, and only know Catholicity to despise it. Many of them have not even received baptism. There are a good number of Irishmen among them, all of who ask for the priest. Our good missionaries gladly accede to their desires; and many souls who have long been estranged from God are reconciled and slumber in the sleep of peace.

Nothing is so distressing as a war of this kind; we find the son armed against the father, and brother against brother. A poor young man told one of our Sisters that he had a twin brother on the other side...[8]

The sisters went and worked with almost no food or sleep for a day and a half caring for the soldiers as they came into the hospital. When the sick men were settled, the sisters returned to Charity Hospital.

Surgeon General Hammond sent them a telegram saying that their help hadn't been needed for a short time but for an unknown length of time because the hospital was Marine Hospital was going to continue to be used. The three sisters returned and remained at the Marine Hospital until the end of the war.

This left Sister Regina shorthanded at Charity Hospital, but somehow the sisters managed. Between 1862 and 1865, the 540-bed hospital had 22,268 patients. This was at a time when hospital stays could last months. The patients also came in waves following a battle, which would overwhelm the available beds and most of the floor space.[9]

A few days later, the Provost Marshal requested that the sister servant of St. Louis Hospital send sisters to the Gratiot and Myrtle Street Prisons. When Sisters Othelia Marshall, Mary Agnes Kelley, Melania Fischer, and Florence O'Hara first arrived, the patients refused their assistance, due to anti-Catholic prejudice. "Prejudice greeted us everywhere. The patients would not even speak to us, though bereft of every consolation of soul and body. However, we were not discouraged but persevered in our work of mercy,"[10] one sister wrote.

One of the doctors commented that "the only kindness received in the prisons has been from Catholics and Sisters of Charity."[11]

The sisters prepared food for the prisoners at their hospital and brought it to the prisons at noon each day. The food helped win the prisoners over so that they accepted the sisters. One sister wrote:

Now that they looked on us with confidence, they would flock to us like children around a mother, to make known to us their little wants, which Providence never failed to supply to their great astonishment. They would frequently ask us how we could provide for so many. We replied that our Lord made the provision.[12]

The sisters had a calming effect on the men at the prison. "A check or two from a sister would be enough so that an improper word was rarely heard. Others who loved their glass of liquor, feared only the sisters knowing it," wrote one sister.[13]

In the Second Battle of Bull Run, August 29 and 30, 1862, the Confederate Army defeated the Union Army once again, and the Union forces retreated toward Washington where the Daughters of Charity would care for the sick and wounded. Satterlee Hospital and the Daughters of Charity there received 1,500 sick and wounded soldiers, most from the battle. "Many had died on the way from exhaustion, others were in a dying state, so that the chaplain, Father Peter McCrane, was sent to administer the Sacraments,"[14] Sister Mary Gonzaga wrote. The sisters gave the soldiers wines and broth and attempted to alleviate their suffering, but the wards were so crowded that tents were raised to provide space for another 1,000 patients.

In Natchez, Mississippi, one of the Daughters of Charity serving at St. Mary's Asylum wrote, "On the 2nd of September, after three o'clock adoration we heard the first shell booming over our heads, without a moment's warning. The reality seemed to fill everyone with consternation. The scene that followed is beyond description. Women and children rushing through the streets screaming in terror."[15]

Many of them rushed to the orphanage seeking safety within its walls and believing that the shells would not fall on a place where God's work was being done. Others wanted to be baptized or have their confessions heard so that they could die in peace. The sister wrote:

I can never forget the anguish I felt at the sight of mothers with infants in their arms, begging us to preserve the lives of their infants, without a seeming thought about their own safety. At the sound of the first shell our good bishop hastened to the asylum, to assist us in placing the children out of danger of the shells about five miles beyond the city.[16]

Those who believed that God protected the orphanage may have been right, for though a few shells fell in the yard, no one was injured.

No sound was heard but the fervent aspirations of our Holy Bishop, and the suppressed sobs of the small children. Then giving a list blessing, [the bishop] told the sisters to get the children off as soon as possible. When all were in readiness, each child, with a bundle of clothing passed out of the Asylum, with the thought that they were never to enter again its loved walls.[17]

Five of the sisters gathered the children to head out of town to safety. They walked with the infants while the sick children rode in a market wagon. While they were doing this, a shell passed over their heads and landed some distance off, but it did not explode. "Our poor children had to run five miles without resting, so great was the danger,"[18] one sister wrote.

The five Daughters of Charity and children would live in the countryside for weeks before returning to Natchez. Meanwhile, three days after the bombardment, three sisters from St. Mary's Asylum were assigned to Monroe, Louisiana, at the request of General Albert Gallatin Blanchard, who commanded in Monroe and was also a Catholic.

Sister Geraldine Murphy, Sister Emerita Quinlan, and Sister Vincentia Conway left Natchez immediately because it was rumored a federal gunboat was approaching the city, which would have forced the city into a barricade situation.

They crossed the Mississippi River about 11 p.m. and traveled for two more days. William Henry Elder, bishop of Natchez and the pastor of Monroe, crossed on the skiff with the sisters and rode with them in the ambulances.[19] The sisters reached Monroe on September 8, where they had charge of the hospital in the city.

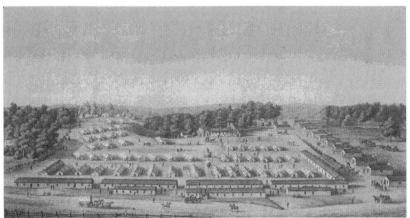

Cliffburne Hospital in Washington D.C. was one of the many hospitals where the Daughters of Charity administered and nursed. Courtesy of the Library of Congress.

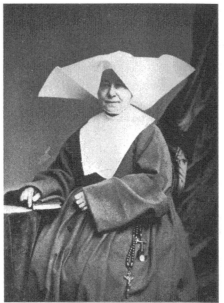

Sister Mary Gonzaga Grace ran Satterlee Hospital in Philadelphia, Pa. during the Civil War. Scanned from *Angels of the Battlefield.* (above) Lincoln Hospital in Washington D.C. during the Civil War. Courtesy of the Library of Congress. (below).

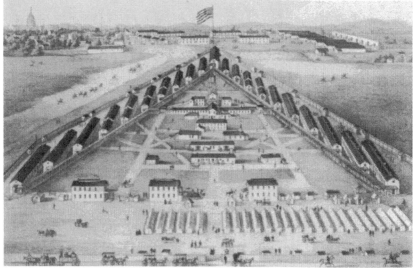

CHAPTER 11
Antietam

"I cannot tell you what a strange impression your presence give me, sad and joyful at the same time, for I fear you are here only in the hope of alleviating our distress."

Protestant minister
at Antietam

As the Confederate Army crossed the Potomac River and marched north in September 1862, it soon became apparent they were heading towards Frederick, Maryland, in the center of the state.

"The present seems to be the most propitious time since the commencement of the war for the Confederate army to enter Maryland," General Robert E. Lee wrote on September 3.[1]

After his victory at the Second Battle of Bull Run at the end of August, Lee moved his army into Maryland with the intention of securing a victory in the North. He wanted to keep his army on the offensive and influence the fall elections in the North so that congressmen and senators willing to recognize the Confederate States of America might be elected. Also, Lee needed supplies for his army that the South was running out of.

"This Morning our town is in a Small Commotion. The report is that Stonewall Jackson has Crossed the Potomack at Nolands Ferry (12 or 14 miles South of this place) with 12,000 men,"[2] Frederick citizen Jacob Engelbrecht wrote in his diary on September 5.

Before the Confederate Army even arrived, citizens of Frederick were seeing refugees flow into the city from the south into Frederick. Even as many people rode and walked from the south, many city residents were heading further north away from the city. "General consternation and a grand stampede of loyal citizens ensured," one person reported.[3]

Patients from the United States Military Hospital where the Daughters of Charity had been working since June 4 were among those evacuated from the city.

As the Confederate Army approached on September 5, the sisters were awakened during the evening and told they had to evacuate the patients from the hospital.

Besides having a hospital in the city, there was also a Union supply depot in the city, which would have been an attractive target for the Confederate Army. Captain William Faithful of the 1st Maryland Regiment, Potomac Home Brigade received orders to drive off the horses and remove or destroy all federal property to keep it from falling into Confederate hands.

"We succeeded in getting off all the most valuable hospital stores in wagons and ambulances, together with about three hundred convalescents from the hospital, to a place of safety in Pennsylvania. After having sent all the most valuable stores by all availing means at hand, we set about destroying by fire the remains," Faithful reported.[4] The flames were said to be seen miles away.

The sisters had gone to bed, but the sister in charge hurried into their room and woke them. They were told that the Confederate Army was in Maryland. All the patients who could be evacuated were leaving as well as the male attendants and any male employees at the hospital. The hospital was expected to be emptied within an hour.

"Imagine our feelings at such news! The hour passed like a flash; the soldiers had all disappeared except a few badly wounded, who could not be removed. The signal was given and in a few moments we beheld the entire city, as it were, enveloped in flames and smoke, so great was the conflagration of the military stores. O, my God! May we never again behold such a sight," Sister Matilda wrote. The doctors who remained behind to care for those soldiers too sick to be moved brought their instruments and other items of value to the sisters for safekeeping, not only trusting the sisters with their safeguarding but knowing they would not be searched or robbed by the Confederate Army.[5]

Catherine Markell was a Frederick resident who watched the Union troops leave Frederick from her roof. She wrote, "Rumors of the approach of the Confederate Army—Federals are burning their stores and 'Skedaddling.' We stayed on the roof of the house until after midnight. Saw the sick from the Barrick hospital straggling, with bandaged heads, etc., toward Pa."[6]

The next morning dawned quietly. Few remained on the hospital grounds, and those that did awaited the inevitable coming of the invading army. One sick soldier told the sisters, "Oh, Sisters, did you stay to [take] care of us? We thought you would have gone, and then what would have become of us?"

Later that morning, two Confederate cavalrymen galloped into the town shouting, "Jefferson Davis!" and "The time of your delivery has come!" Colonel Bradley Johnson and 150 horsemen soon followed. Military bands played "Maryland, My Maryland" and "Dixie" as the Southern troops marched into Frederick. General Stonewall Jackson's advance force of 5,000 men marched up Market Street and camped on the north side of town.[7]

However, the enthusiastic response the Confederate army had expected from residents was not to be seen. "We were rather disappointed at our reception, which was decidedly cool. This wasn't what we expected...There was positively no enthusiasm, no cheers, no waving handkerchiefs and flags—instead a death-like silence—some houses were closed tight, as if some public calamity had taken place," wrote Confederate infantryman Alexander Hunter.[8]

At the hospital, a Confederate officer demanded that the doctors surrender the facility to the Confederate Army, which they did. The Confederate soldiers accepted the surrender and brought about 400 of their own sick and wounded into the hospital.

The Daughters of Charity who were working at the hospital were not only shocked at the condition of the men who were brought in for their care but also at the state of those who were bringing them to the hospital. The soldiers told the sisters they had survived on green corn for the previous two weeks. They were "young and old men, with boys who seemed like mere children, emaciated with hunger and covered with tattered rags that gave them more the appearance of dead men than living ones."[9]

The sisters had begun to administer to the ill Confederates when the chief surgeon told them that as employees of the Union government, they couldn't give aid to the Confederates soldiers.[10]

Part of the problem the sisters faced was that the Maryland General Assembly had passed a treason bill in the spring. The new law made it illegal for state and federal workers to provide aid and comfort to the enemy. Since the Daughters of Charity who served in the war were considered federal employees, even if many of them volunteered their services,[11] they could not give aid to the Confederate soldiers, or they would find themselves arrested and unable to provide assistance to anyone, Confederate or Union. For eight days, the sisters could do nothing to ease the Confederates' suffering.

Townspeople weren't so bound, and they provided cakes to the soldiers, but in some cases, the fatty foods were too much for the starving men and proved fatal.[12] Young men in the nearby Jesuit novitiate volunteered to nurse the sick and "happily their services were accepted by the U.S. Surgeon who fixed accommodations for them to stay at the barracks," one of the sisters wrote.[13]

On September 11, two sisters got a pass from General Lee to travel to Emmitsburg to inform their superiors of the situation in Frederick.

In the meantime, Major General George B. McClellan had gathered the Army of the Potomac and headed after the Confederate Army. This led to the army leaving Frederick and heading west over South Mountain. By the time the sisters returned from Emmitsburg, Frederick had been abandoned by the Confederates. At that point, the doctors made no distinction between Union and Confederate soldiers and helped anyone who needed it.[14]

One sister wrote that the soldiers wrote that the soldiers "lay side by side so that we had it in our power to give them equal attention. It was truly edifying to see the patience and harmony that reigned among them. Sometimes they would say, 'Sister we are not enemies except on the battlefield.'"[15]

That would happen soon enough.

General McClellan caught up with General Lee's army on South Mountain, and the two armies began fighting. The Confederate Army tried to block the Union at the mountain passes without success. McClellan's men pushed through the passes and over the mountain.

The Confederate Army retreated to the west, and Lee considered heading south. But with General Stonewall Jackson's capture of Harpers Ferry on September 15, General Lee decided to make a stand at Sharpsburg.

On September 17, a foggy morning, cannons and rifle fire erupted between the towns of Boonsboro and Sharpsburg. So began a twelve-hour battle that would become the deadliest single day for America. Nearly 100,000 soldiers would eventually fight that day, and by day's end, nearly 23,000 would be casualties.

The following day began the work to save the wounded and bury the dead.

Maryland authorities had already requested help from the Daughters of Charity to help with the wounded on the day of the battle. "The people of the area were asked to help the Confederate soldiers, and the Sisters and people of Emmitsburg collected clothing, provisions, remedies, and money."[16]

Father Edward Smith, C.M., a pastor in Emmitsburg, drove two sisters to Boonsboro in a wagon. They arrived at twilight after the battle's end and found four hospitals for Union wounded and three for Confederate wounded. "But as the fighting had

James Rada, Jr.

been over twelve or fifteen miles space, the towns of Boonsboro and Sharpsburg were hospitals," wrote Sister Matilda Coskery.[17]

When the Daughters of Charity arrived, two Union officers recognized the sisters by their cornettes and one said, "Ah, there come the Sisters of Charity; now the poor men will be equally cared for."[18]

The sisters headed immediately to the battlefield to search for wounded among the many dead bodies. On their way there they found all the houses and barns being used as hospitals with the wooden fencing, where there was still any left, draped with bloody clothing. The wounded lay on the ground with only a bit of straw for a mattress. If they were lucky, a blanket might have been stretched out on sticks driven into the ground to provide shade. Otherwise, they had had no protection from the sun during the day as they suffered from their wounds.[19]

The sisters set about to improve the conditions of the injured by distributing the goods they had brought with them. Sister Matilda wrote of the soldiers, "Unable to move or change their position, every filth surrounded them; add to this, vermin, maggots and stench. Bullets could be gathered from between them, that lay scattered around."[20]

This would have been particularly troubling to her because she had repeatedly written about the need for cleanliness not only of the patients but also of the utensils and medical instruments that touched the patient and the sick room that surrounded him.[21]

The wounded were already being transferred to hospitals, not only in the small village of Boonsboro but in the larger cities of Frederick and Hagerstown as well.

All around them, the Daughters of Charity saw devastation. The crops had been trampled, the fences had been used for fuel, livestock had disappeared, and even the dogs were either killed or had fled from the appalling scene. Sister Matilda wrote of the scene:

…that on no battlefield during the war were any of those

128

carrier (sic) birds seen, not even a crow; though piles of dead horses lay here and there, some half-burned from efforts made to consume them by lighting fence rails on them—but these seems rather to add to the foulness of the atmosphere than to help purify it.[22]

When the supplies the sisters had brought with them were used up, they told one surgeon, "We are sorry. We have nothing to offer you but poor sympathy."

"Oh," replied the surgeon, "the sympathy of a Sister of Charity is a great boon to our soldiers at any time."[23]

The sisters found themselves "in constant danger from bomb shells which had not exploded and which only required a slight jar to burst. The ground was covered with these, and it was hard to distinguish them when the carriage wheels were rolling over straw and dry leaves."[24]

The battle's 23,000 casualties nearly overwhelmed the sisters' ability to help them. Someone always seemed to need their attention. No matter how fast they were able to offer care to one soldier, there were always two more waiting.

With so much death around them, the sisters had little patience for anyone trying to add more. At one point, a Union steward and Confederate surgeon got into an argument on the battlefield that escalated to the point that one challenged the other to a fight to the death on the battlefield that was already saturated with blood. As both men left to duel, yelling at each other, one of the sisters followed. She dressed them down and took their pistols from them. Ashamed, the men returned to their posts and resumed their work.[25]

The sisters approached one mortally wounded soldier in a wagon shed and were told by an officer that the man had been a hero as a flag bearer during the fighting.

"I fear the man is dying rapidly; come to him," the officer said. "He has been so valiant that I wish to let his wife know that the Sisters of Charity were with him in his last moments."

And so the sisters remained with him. Father Smith was brought in to give the man last rites. With the sisters near, the soldier faced his death with a courage matched by what he had shown in battle.[26]

The Union medical director sought to thank the sister for coming to the aid of the soldiers and asked them to dine with him at dinner. The sisters tried to decline, but the officer wouldn't take "no" for an answer. So they joined him at his dinner table and ate "spoiled pork and war biscuit, the dinner, with tea in bowls large enough for bleeding purposes, and much we feared they were used for that purpose!" Sister Matilda wrote. Instead, the sisters withdrew some of the provisions they had brought and ate unspoiled food.[27]

Following the meal, "Night drove us to our lodgings in the town before we were ready for it but returning to the same field the next morning, those we had assisted the day previous, were consigned to the earth; and they that could not consent yesterday to receive baptism, now eagerly received it," Sister Matilda wrote.[28]

One of the men "consigned to the earth" was the flag bearer who the Daughters of Charity had seen die the day before. Besides the sisters and Father Smith, about ten others attended the service.

During the funeral, a group of horsemen approached the sisters and removed their hats.

"I am General McClellan, and I am happy and proud to see the Sisters of Charity with these poor men. How many are here?" the general asked.

"Two," one of the sisters answered. "We came here to bring relief to the suffering, and we return in a day or so."

"Oh, why can we not have more here? I would like to see fifty sisters ministering to the poor sufferers. Who shall I address for this purpose?"

Father Smith supplied the general with a name and address where the request could be sent. Then McClellan asked after the welfare of the flag bearer.

When he was told that the flag bearer was about to be buried, McClellan joined in the funeral procession.[29]

Though the Daughters of Charity intended to stay only a few days, the wound up staying three weeks, washing, dressing wounds, baptizing, feeding and praying for thousands of wounded men.

As the battlefield has often proven true the old saying, "Necessity is the mother of invention," so it was in the Civil War. One of the improvements brought about by the war came at Antietam.

The Army of the Potomac's medical director, Jonathan Letterman, had only been in the position since earlier that summer. He was a graduate of Jefferson Medical College in Philadelphia. One of his first changes to the army was to take control of the ambulance wagons from the Quartermaster Department and assign it to the Medical Department. As had been seen during earlier battles, ambulance drivers would often refuse to take orders from doctors even if it was a request to help fallen soldiers. Letterman also created a standardized medical wagon for each regiment.

After Antietam, Letterman developed the Letterman Ambulance Plan that was used following the battle. Under the plan, a division's ambulances moved together. Each ambulance had a mounted line sergeant, two stretcher bearers, and a driver. These ambulances would bring the wounded from the battlefield to a dressing station and then to a field hospital.

Previously men had been assigned to ambulance duty as the need arose. However, these tended to be men who weren't good soldiers and were little better as battlefield medics. They had been known to get drunk while on the job or to hide when the fighting began, leaving their wounded comrades on the field.

The new ambulance system proved a success at Antietam and got a lot of wounded men to the medical care they needed.

James Rada, Jr.

In Frederick, where the Daughters of Charity were once again able to administer to both Union and Confederate soldiers, the United States Hospital filled quickly with wounded from the battle. The U.S. government ordered churches and other buildings in the city turned into hospitals. The Jesuit Novitiate and Visitation Academy were among them.

"Here was a scene of carnage not to be described; the two armies who had so exultingly passed our windows but a few days before, now returned weltering in each other's gore. What a reflection for the human mind! Could man only comprehend the horrors of Fratricidal War, it would be enough to prevent him from engaging in it ever!" one of the Daughters of Charity wrote.[30]

For the next six weeks, the sisters worked with little rest as they worked to care for the patients.

More help was requested from Emmitsburg, but the Superiors at St. Joseph's could only send a few more sisters to help with the need at that time.

In September, Father Burlando removed the sisters from the military transports they had been serving on because they had no opportunity to attend Mass even when the ships were in port.

Those floating hospitals were, however, very frightful: more than four or five hundred sick and wounded lay heaped on one another; the bottom, middle and hold of the ships were filled with sufferers. Willingly would we have continued our services, but our Sisters were deprived of all spiritual assistance; no mass or communion; even when they entered the port, it was hard for them to go to church, either because they did not know where there was one, or because the distance would not allow them. We were therefore obliged to remove and place them in the organized hospitals on land, where they can at least rely on the assistance of a priest.[31]

The sisters were reassigned to serve at locations where the Council of St. Joseph's saw the greatest need, such as Point Lookout.

In Washington City, the work of the sisters continued in Eckington Military Hospital. The hospital was in the northwest quadrant of the city South of Prospect Hill and Glenwood Cemeteries in the country home of Joseph Gales, Jr., the owner of the *National Intelligencer* newspaper. Gales had also been the mayor of Washington from 1827 to 1830. The two-story house sat on top of a hill. The doctor in charge was Dr. W.W. Keen who had graduated medical school in March 1861, joined the army in May 1861 and was put in charge of Eckington Military Hospital that same month.[32]

The hospital was large enough to hold about 400 patients who were under the care of nine sisters who had "charge of distributing the medicines, of superintending the wards and preserving good order and cleanliness, and in general of everything concerning the welfare of the sick."[33]

This was the nicer hospital compared to the Cliffburne Hospital also in Washington City on Meridian Hill. There thirteen sisters cared for 1,200 soldiers in a tent-and-shed hospital.

As winter came on, it turned out to be a harsh one in central Virginia. In Danville, the railroad workshops had been converted into a hospital during the summer that was capable of holding 500 patients. "The location is excellent for the purpose, being upon the banks of the river, free from the unhealthy atmosphere of the city, and commanding a continual current of pure air, fresh from the clouds and forests," reported the *Richmond Enquirer*.[34] What it wasn't capable of holding was heat. The low temperatures caused the patients to all be moved to Lynchburg so that they would not suffer from hypothermia.

Five Daughters of Charity followed their 1,000 patients in the move and remained at the hospital in Ferguson's Tobacco Factory in Lynchburg for three years until the end of the war. The conditions in the hospital were still not the best, though they were better than they had been in Danville, according to Sister Angela Heath. She wrote:

> The persons who were in charge, had a very good will, but not the means of carrying it out, and although the fund was ample, the poor patients were half starved, owing entirely to the mismanagement.
>
> To give you an idea of the care the sick had received, it will be sufficient to say that, though the whole establishment had been cleaned up for our reception some of the sisters swept up the vermin on the dustpan.[35]

In early November, the Council of St. Joseph's assigned another sister to Satterlee Hospital. Two more sisters would be sent there in December. In the three years that the Daughters of Charity nursed at Satterlee, ninety-one Daughters of Charity served here, though no more than forty-three at any one time.

During May of 1864, the Satterlee Hospital personnel would treat more than 12,000 patients, of which only 260 died. This was a miraculous feat at a time when more soldiers died from disease and infection than wounds. Sister Mary Gonzaga Grace wrote of what the hospital was like that month:

> We have now nearly three thousand four hundred patients in our Hospital. Indeed, it is as if we were in the midst of a little city. Everywhere we turn we meet crowds of the maimed, the lame and the blind, going through the corridors and yards as best they can. The wards are quickly filling up with rows of beds in the centre, as new arrivals are coming in every day from the recent battles.[36]

In the Confederate States of America, the value of the female nurses was measured and found to be a great boon to a soldier's health and chances of recovery. The *Galveston Weekly News* reported on a debate in the Confederate Senate as to whether female nurses should be used in the hospitals in the Confederate States.

Senator Thomas Semmes of Louisiana stood before his colleagues and reported to them that the mortality rate in Clopton Hospital in Richmond, which used female nurses, was two percent. The death rate at the Francis de Sales Hospital that the Daughters of Charity ran was three percent. However, in hospitals where there were no female nurses, the average mortality rate was ten percent.[37]

On November 14, General Ambrose Burnside, newly commanding the Army of the Potomac sent a corps to occupy Falmouth, Virginia, and followed shortly after that with his entire army. The army stalled temporarily at the Rappahannock River waiting for supplies to build bridges. Even after they crossed the river on pontoon bridges on December 11, Burnside did not engage the Confederate Army.

General Lee took advantage of the delay and took the heights behind Fredericksburg. When Burnside did decide to engage the Confederates, they were well entrenched on the high ground.

The casualties were enormous. Of the more than 172,000 men involved in the battle, there were nearly 18,000 casualties. The Union Army had the heaviest losses with 13,353 out of 100,007 soldiers engaged.

Following the battle, the Daughters of Charity began their work caring for more than 1,600 wounded. The poet Walt Whitman was a Civil War nurse who described the battlefield at Fredericksburg as a "butcher's shambles" and a field hospital:

O well it is their mothers, their sisters cannot see them— cannot conceive, and never conceiv'd, these things. One man is shot by a shell, both in the arm and leg—both are amputated—there lie the rejected members. Some have their legs blown off—some bullets through the breast—

James Rada, Jr.

some indescribably horrid wounds in the face or head, all mutilated, sickening, torn, gouged out—some in the abdomen—some mere boys…the surgeons use them just the same.[38]

Many of the wounded had further complications caused by vermin carrying diseases and attacking wounds. The sisters remained at the field hospital at Fredericksburg for three weeks until the wounded could be moved to regular hospitals.[39]

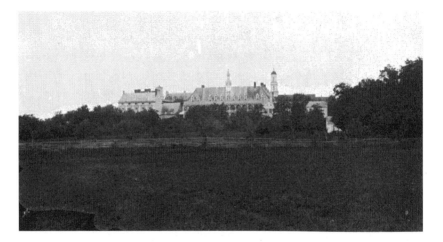

A view of St. Joseph's Academy during the Civil War. The Union Army would camp in the fields around college in the days before the Battle of Gettysburg. Courtesy of the Library of Congress.

CHAPTER 12
Daughters of Charity Invaded

"A Protestant minister who was a constant visitor at the hospital asked me if I was ever tired. I told him I was, very often. 'You must get a large salary for what you do' I told him no less than the Kingdom of Heaven."

Sister Rose Noyland
Daughter of Charity

At the very beginning of 1863, it appeared that the Union Army may have turned a corner in its war efforts. On New Year's Day, President Lincoln issued the Emancipation Proclamation that freed all slaves in states that were in rebellion against the United States. It had little effect on the daily lives of slaves since the Confederate States of America didn't recognize the United States of America's authority over it, nor did it free the slaves in the Union, but it gave the Union the moral upper hand in the war. On the following day, the Union Army emerged victorious from the Battle of Murfreesboro in Tennessee.

The Daughters of Charity continued their work among the sick and wounded on both sides of the conflict. On January 8, a patient in the military hospital at Monroe, Louisiana, was upset that Sister Emerita Quinlan wasn't giving him special attention. The area had become overcrowded as residents and soldiers had fled the Union invasion of New Orleans in 1862. Although they had left New Orleans and the surrounding region, the sick and wounded still needed care and so hospitals had been set up.

As she walked by his bed one time, she heard him curse at

her. Sister Emerita Quinlan stopped and told him that she didn't appreciate him using vulgar language around her. He apologized, and she continued on with her arms full of bottles.

She stopped to talk to another patient who was recovering from his wounds, and she felt the urge to turn around. She did so and saw the man she had just corrected reach his hand into his coat, draw a pistol and fire it at her. The bullet passed through her cornette within a couple of inches of her forehead.[1]

The poor man whom she was addressing thought he was wounded again. He jumped and clapped his hands on his old wound as if to assure himself of its escape from harm. Sister still held her bottles and made her way through the cloud of smoke caused by the firing of the pistol and the crowd that gathered at its report. The man was arrested, but at sister's request, he was released.[2]

The shooter said it had been an accident. He was a gambler, and he had loaded to the pistol to shoot an officer in town.[3]

Further north along the Mississippi River, St. Louis was inundated with wounded soldiers after battles. Hospital steamboats would pick up patients from battlefields, treat them and take them to St. Louis for further treatment and recuperation there. More than 800 wounded were known to arrive in the city in a single day.

Union soldiers were treated at the city hospital or the Jefferson Barracks, which had been converted into a hospital for 3,000 patients.

The Daughters of Charity ran DePaul Hospital in St. Louis, which began as the St. Louis Mullanphy Hospital in 1828. It was established in the home of John Mullanphy on Spruce Street and was the first Catholic hospital in the United States and the first hospital west of Mississippi.

St. Louis, like many other communities, had established a sanitary commission to help in the war effort. St. Louis' group was called the Western Sanitary Commission. The women who were members made bandages, scraped lint and sent food to army hospitals.

The Western Sanitary Commission asked for the help of the Daughters of Charity on January 14 to care for the Confederate prisoners of war. The Council of St. Joseph's named Sister Othelia Marshall as the procuratrix and a sister already at the hospital to care for the prisoners of war.[4]

Further east, five sisters left Richmond for Marietta, Georgia, on February 24. They were met with amazement at many of the places they stopped on their journey south. At one stop, the sisters had to wait two hours for a train. They sat on the benches quietly as the other passengers gathered around the stove to warm themselves and steal glances at the sisters.

"Who are they?"

"Are they men or women?"

"Oh, what a strange uniform this company has adopted."

"Surely the enemy will run from them."

Once or twice the crowd jostled the sisters "as though to see whether they were human beings or not."

One of the sisters spoke to one of the women on the platform and delighted the crowd. They clapped their hands and shouted, "She spoke! She spoke!"[5]

At one town, the sisters sought out the local Catholic priest for help in finding a place to stay for the night. The priest had never seen a Daughter of Charity with their white cornettes and expressed skepticism that they were Catholic sisters.

Finally, he agreed to take them to the home of the Sisters of Mercy, the order of Catholic sisters in the city. The Mother at the Sisters of Mercy's home recognized the Daughters of Charity and welcomed them into the house. Upon confirmation of their identity, the relieved priest admitted that he had thought they were imposters.[6]

Further along in their journey, the sisters' train came to a sudden stop, throwing some passengers off balance. One panicked passenger shouted that the train had fallen through a bridge and crashed into a river. The passengers scrambled to get off the train, but the sisters remained calm. Soon it was discovered that their train hadn't been involved in an accident, but another train that had been coming in the opposite direction had had an accident. Some passengers took up torches to go and help passengers in the other train.

Two of the sisters were able to cross the bridge. Once on the other side, they began to help the wounded from the other train. Luckily, no one had been killed or severely wounded.[7]

The sisters reached the nearest town around midnight but found no food available. They continued to work to help the injured by feeding them from the food they carried in their basket. One sister wrote, "Fortunately, our little basket prepared for five Sisters afforded some support, but by this time our band had increased to eleven. These and several strangers with whom we also shared, ate and truly our basket was still full."[8]

In all, it took the sisters three days to get to Marietta and once there, they went to work in one of the many hospitals there including the hotel, many of the churches and large houses. For five weeks they attended to the sick and wounded while not being able to attend Mass. Two sisters made the trip to Atlanta to plead with army officials and church representatives to conduct Mass on Easter Sunday. However, the hospital was moved to Atlanta before a chaplain could be assigned.[9]

The sisters followed the hospital patients and arrived in Atlanta on May 24. They found conditions there nearly the opposite of what they had been in Marietta. Almost all of the houses in Atlanta were filled with sick and wounded. The only place that could be found for the sisters to stay was in tents. Their first charges were about 500 soldiers who were also housed tents, and the number of patients continued to grow daily.

Eventually, a small two-room log cabin was found for the sisters, but it was not much better than their tent. "The mice ran over us at night and the rain was so constant through the day that our umbrellas were always in their hands,"[10] wrote one sister.

While in Atlanta, an officer with a bias against Catholics observed the Daughters of Charity and took notes on the sisters' conduct and what they said. The sisters didn't mind their shadow and went about their duties as usual. One sister later wrote, "He did not proceed very far before he asked for a book that would tell him of our Faith. The result was his own fervent entrance into that church he had so much despised."[11]

In another example of how the service of the Daughters of Charity softened hearts prejudiced against Catholics, one angry patient continued to be rude to the sisters despite being shown only kindness.

Finally, a sister asked the man, "Have I pained you? I know I am too rough. Pardon me this time, and I will try to spare you pain again, for I would rather lessen than augment distress in this hour of misery."

The man began crying. "My heart is indeed pained at my ingratitude towards you, for I have received nothing less than maternal care from you, and I have received it in anger. Do pardon me. I declare I am forced to respect your patience and charity. When I came into this hospital and found that the Sisters were the nurses my heart was filled with hatred. My mind was filled with prejudice—a prejudice which I confess was inherited from those nearest and dearest to me. I did not believe that anything good could come from the Sisters. But now I see my mistake all too clearly, and in seeing it, I recognize the unintentional blackness of my own heart.

"I have seen the Sisters in their true light. I see their gentleness, their humility, their daily—aye, their hourly sacrifices, their untiring work for others; in a word, their great love for humanity. Forgive me if you can."

After such a heartfelt apology, the sister quickly forgave the man. Helping him became a pleasant experience rather than a chore.[12]

James Rada, Jr.

* * *

In Washington, President Abraham Lincoln appointed General Joseph Hooker to command of the Army of the Potomac. Hooker did so and took his army of 115,000 soldiers to converge on Chancellorsville, Virginia. Hooker expected General Robert E. Lee to retreat in the face of an army nearly twice the size of his.

Instead of retreating, Lee divided his army, leaving one group to protect Fredericksburg while the rest moved to confront the Union army.

The van of Hooker's men clashed with the Confederates on May 1, 1865. Hooker pulled back to Chancellorsville near the Wilderness, a dense wood. He hoped that the dense undergrowth of the Wilderness would cause the Confederates problems if they attacked.

Lee divided his men again. He left two divisions to hold Hooker's attention while General Stonewall Jackson took the bulk of the army across the Union line to a position near the Union Army's exposed right flank on May 2. His men struck two hours before dusk, catching the Union army in their camp.

The Confederates stopped fighting around 9 p.m. when things became too confused in the dense underbrush. Jackson himself was a victim of the confusion. Riding near the front lines to reconnoiter, a Confederate soldier accidentally shot him in the arm severely wounding him. Surgeons amputated the arm later that night.

The following day, General J.E.B. Stuart assumed command in place of the wounded General Jackson. He attempted to reunite his men with those of Lee. Hooker fought back hard but was forced to give ground.

The Confederate Army was converging on Chancellorsville and Hooker when a message from General Jubal Early reached Lee saying the Union Army had broken through the Confederate line at Fredericksburg.

Lee reinforced his men at Fredericksburg and forced the Un-

142

ion Army to retreat across the Rappahannock River. When he returned to Chancellorsville, Hooker had also taken his men across the river.

The result of the battle was 14,000 Confederate casualties and 17,000 casualties on the Union side. Among the Confederate casualties was Jackson who died of pneumonia on May 10 while recuperating from the amputation of his arm.

Further south, Union General Ulysses S. Grant attacked Vicksburg, Mississippi, on May 19 and 22. He had been trying to take the city for a year, but once again both attacks were repulsed due to the strength of the miles of defensive lines around the city. Because of this, Grant decided to put the city under siege.

By June, General Lee had decided to go on the offensive and take the war into the North into Maryland once again. Mother Ann Simeon wrote to the Mother Elizabeth Montcellet in France about the push north.

Our good Father Burlando has been obliged to leave us again to go to Saint Louis. Since his departure, the Confederate Army has gained ground, and is advancing upon us; it is already in our poor little Maryland, at twenty-two miles from the Central House. Frederick, which is quite near us, was taken without any bloodshed, but we expect a terrible battle soon; perhaps it is even now going on. We are praying heartily for peace, and we have had perpetual adoration during the last three days. We fear, my Most Honored Mother, that our prized intercourse with you will be interupted for a time. Do not forget before God your poor Daughters of the United States.[13]

Emmitsburg also had other worries closer to home. Around 11 p.m. on Monday night, June 15, flames took hold of the Beam and Guthrie Livery Stable at Emmitsburg. "People in the country heard the church bells ring; some came within a mile of town, looking at the blazing houses, but feared to come in, as they thought the rebel army had fired it, as they had done Chambersburg."[14]

From the Beam and Guthrie Livery Stable, the fire jumped the alley and consumed the northwest corner of the town square from the back. From there, it spread east and southeast, and as a result of the prevailing northwest winds that night, it worked its way down Main Street on both sides.

Lawrence Owen, an Emmitsburg shoemaker, was among the first to lose his home. As the fire grew, it spread to many more. Residents gave up trying to save their homes and tried to get the valuables and furniture outside. Unfortunately, many of the homes they moved items to also burned.

The Wiles' City Hotel, a four-story structure built only four years previously, was the last building to burn. The structure survived but with $10,000 in damage, a fortune in those days.[15]

Townspeople and students from Mount Saint Mary's College and Seminary began their desperate efforts to quench the flames. Word of the fire reached the college around midnight. The president of the school, Rev. John McCloskey woke the older boys and college employees. They rode into Emmitsburg, still tired, and began working the water pumps and filling tubs and the tank for the pumper with water.[16]

The townspeople placed wet blankets on the roof of the Donohue house on the southwest corner of the town square, the only corner of the square that didn't burn. The dampness kept the flames from spreading to the building and allowed the townspeople and college students time to finally put the fire out around 7 a.m.

By the time the flames sputtered out, twenty-eight houses and nine businesses were damaged or destroyed. Three of the four corners of the town square were black with fire, and all four of the four blocks to the east of the square were fire damaged. Other reports put the number of damaged buildings at fifty and half of the town destroyed. In actuality, probably about a quarter of the town burned, based on a population of slightly less than 1,000.[17]

As the losses were tallied from what was called "the most serious calamity in the history of the town," 189 people, about twenty percent of Emmitsburg's population, had lost homes, furnishings, farm animals, business goods and/or businesses. Forty-two property owners totaled their losses at $82,000 or twenty-two percent of the value of all the property owned by citizens in Emmitsburg in 1860.[18]

Mother Ann Simeon offered the White House to the people who had been left homeless after the fire and offered help to others.[19] Dr. William Patterson and his family were among those who lost their homes in the fire and took the Daughters of Charity up on their offer. The Pattersons actually wound up residing in the White House for the rest of Dr. Patterson's life.

Rumors that Confederate sympathizers had started the fire spread as quickly as the fire. However, Eli Smith was arrested and jailed for causing the fire, and he was not known to be a sympathizer.[20]

Mother Ann Simeon shared an apartment with her secretary Sister Marie Louise Caulfield at St. Joseph's Academy. Their two rooms in the Gothic Building were connected by double doors that remained open. The corner apartment had a clear, unobstructed view of the surrounding countryside through the Southern and western windows.

On Saturday night, June 27, Mother Ann Simeon had already turned in, but Sister Marie Louise was still awake when she heard unfamiliar sounds outside the building. As the noises seemed to draw closer, she made out the neighing of horses among them.

She rose from her bed and looked outside. She saw lights flashing on and off on a hill near the end of the toll gate that was nearby. With the rumors of approaching armies that had been circulating throughout the town, Sister Marie Louise realized that

James Rada, Jr.

it was no longer a rumor.

She gently shook Mother Ann Simeon awake and told her what she had seen. The two women dressed and slipped quietly outside into the darkness. They walked to another building on the campus and climbed an exterior staircase to the second floor of the building.

By this time, they were no longer alone in their journey. Other sisters, awakened by the sound of the approaching army, had also come outside to investigate. The sisters moved through the music rooms of the second floor of the building and climbed another staircase, in this case an interior one, to the cupola on the roof of the square Bruté Building, dedicated to the memory of Father Simon Bruté, who had been a spiritual director and chaplain to the Sisters of Charity beginning in 1818 until 1834. The sisters taught astronomy classes from the cupola because it afforded the best view of the sky on the campus.

They stood in the darkness of the night watching the lights of the approaching army not knowing which army it was. They knew each dot of light represented a handful of men and there were many, many lights. "The field opposite was in fine clover at sunset on Saturday, but when the sun rose on Sunday it was as barren and bare as a board," Sister Marie Louise wrote.[21] The mowing machine that had already been placed in one of the meadows was no longer needed.

The soldiers did not approach the Central House that evening. Instead, they found the overseer for the farm, Joseph Brawner, who lived with his wife in a little house between the academy and the toll gate. The soldiers asked Brawner's permission to camp on the fields that first night.

On Sunday, Brawner was given a receipt that entitled him to be paid for 16,000 pounds of hay that the arriving Army of the Potomac has consumed on the farm.

General Philippe Regis de Trobriand was a French aristocrat who also commanded the Third Brigade of the First Division of the Third Corps. He wrote about his impressions of St. Joseph's the following morning saying:

> I leave it to you to guess if the good sisters were not excited, on seeing the guns moving along under their windows and the regiments, bristling with bayonets, spreading out through their orchards. Nothing like it had ever troubled the calm of this holy retreat. When I arrived at a gallop in front of the principal door, the doorkeeper, who had ventured a few steps outside, completely lost her head. In her fright, she came near being trampled under foot by the horses of my staff, which she must have taken for the horses of the Apocalypse, -- if, indeed, there are any horse in the Apocalypse, of which I am not sure.[22]

The general met Mother Ann Simeon in the parlor and was impressed by her calm and dignity, particularly in the face of the reception he had received earlier. He noted that Mother Ann Simeon grasped the situation and did not object when de Trobiand asked to go to the cupola to observe the surrounding land.

> We reached the belfry by a narrow and winding staircase. I went first. At the noise of my boots sounding on the steps, a rustling of dresses and murmuring of voices were heard above my head. There were eight or ten young nuns, who had mounted up there to enjoy the extraordinary spectacle of guns in battery, of stacked muskets, of sentinels walking back and forth with their arms in hand, of soldiers making coffee in the gardens, of horses ready saddled eating their oats under apple trees; -- all things of which they had not the least idea. We had cut off their retreat, and they were crowded against the windows, like frightened birds, asking Heaven to send them wings with which to fly away.
>
> "Ah! Sisters," I said to them, "I catch you in the very act of curiosity. After all, it is a venial sin, and I am sure

that the very reverend father here present will freely give you absolution therefor."

The poor girls, much embarrassed, looked at each other, not knowing what to reply. The least timid ventured a smile. In their hearts, they were thinking of but one thing: to escape as soon as the officers accompanying me left the way clear.

"Permit me," I said, "to make one request of you. Ask St. Joseph to keep the rebels away from here; for, if they come before I get away, I do not know what will become of your beautiful convent."

They immediately disappeared, crowding each other along the staircase. I have never returned to Emmittsburg; but it would astonish me very little to hear that the two armies had gone to Gettysburg to fight, on account of the miracle performed by St. Joseph, interceding in favor of these pious damsels.[23]

With so many troops encamped on the grounds of their school and Central House, the sisters began to worry that a battle might be fought on their doorsteps.

General Oliver Howard with his staff stayed in the Vincentian residence where Father Burlando lived in Emmitsburg. General Carl Schurz and his officers remained in the White House.

To safeguard the property and sisters at Emmitsburg, the Union generals stationed guards at various points. "Here and there they were dotted standing on guard two hours, fagged out with fatigue, and hungry as wolves," Sister Mary Louise wrote.[24]

The soldiers began asking the sisters for food the day after they began arriving. "The poor fellows looked half-starved,--lank as herrings and barefoot,"[25] Sister Mary Jane Stokes wrote.

The sisters spent their day slicing meat, buttering bread and filling canteens with coffee or milk.

On June 29, D. Agnew, justice of the peace in Emmitsburg, signed a statement of damages the sisters used to get paid for some of the food they provided the army. Though the list did not include the bread and cold meats given the soldiers, it did list: 109 cord wood of fuel at $2.50 a cord, 13.5 tons of hay at $9 a ton and 120 bushels of rye at a dollar a bushel.

Sister Mary Jane Stokes was in charge of the farm. She saw soldiers who were hungry and could not deny them a meal. So the sisters gave freely of what they had, although it quickly diminished their own supplies since feeding an army required much more than feeding a couple hundred sisters and students. As the Daughters of Charity continued to liberally provide all of the soldiers who came asking for food, she realized that the day's supply bread was quickly disappearing. She went to the bakehouse to see if there would be any bread left for the sisters to eat with their meals and was surprised to find that the day's baking hadn't been touched.

> Well, the Sisters were cutting bread, and giving them to eat as fast as they came for it, all the evening, and I was afraid there would be no bread left for the Sisters' supper. However, they had supper and plenty. After supper, I belonged to the kitchen Sisters, I went to Mother Ann Simeon and told her I didn't know what the Sisters would do for breakfast the next morning, for they would have no bread. Then I went to see, and there was the baking of the day was there. I did not see it *multiply, but I did see it there!*[26]

While the sisters took on the job of feeding the soldiers, Fathers Burlando and Gandolfo and another priest from Emmitsburg heard confessions from the Catholic soldiers. "The fathers remained as long as there was a soldier to be heard and invested with a pair of scapulars. Never did we witness such satisfaction as to see those poor men express their hope and confidence in the Mother of God that she would save their souls any way, even if they should fall in the terrible battle that they were facing,"[27] Sis-

149

ter Camilla O'Keefe wrote.

During this time, Father Burlando stayed at St. Joseph's Academy rather than in the house he shared with other priests in Emmitsburg. Besides having his own home occupied by army officers, staying at the academy allowed him to watch over the sisters in his care. Father Burlando slept, when he could sleep, on a couch in the office he used for conducting his duties at the St. Joseph's Central House. However, at the least little sound, he was up and walking the halls fully dressed.

In addition to Father Burlando's caution, two sisters guarded the others each night. One night Sister Marie Louise and another sister were on patrol when suddenly the second sister was startled by the sight of another person in the hall. That person turned out to be Father Burlando on his own patrol of the grounds. They urged him to get some sleep, but he demurred.[28]

Mother Ann Simeon also took care to separate her charges from the soldiers. The doors to the seminary building were kept locked at all times. On one occasion two sisters left on an errand, and when they returned, they found themselves locked out of the building.

Early on June 30, 1863, the order was given to strike camp. "In fifteen minutes, it was done and St. Joseph's Valley relapsed into quiet."[29] Sister Camilla wrote, "Not a vestige of the great Army was to be seen…Glad we were to get rid of them."[30]

While the Daughters of Charity were committed to showing no favoritism in their treatment of the soldiers, the same didn't hold true for the girls who boarded at the academy. Many of them were from Confederate states and were trapped in a country at war with their home states. As the soldiers prepared to leave, one girl climbed into the cupola that towered above the surrounding area and signaled to Confederate scouts where the Union troops were and that they were preparing to leave.[31]

Shortly after the Union Army had headed north out of Emmitsburg when the Confederate Army appeared on the horizon. Though a much smaller army, estimated at only 10,000 men, the soldiers generated much more excitement in the town and at St. Joseph's Academy.[32]

So quick was the switch between the armies during the night that Father Gandolfo did not realize control of the town had changed hands. The next morning, Father Gandolfo came out to St. Joseph's early to say Mass and was halted by Confederate pickets.

Not recognizing the soldiers as Confederate and not knowing the Union Army had moved out, Father Gandolfo said, "But I am going to say Mass at St. Joseph's. We have General Howard at our house."

Though admitting he had housed a Union general didn't help his case, things managed to get straightened out, and he was allowed to continue on his way.[33]

Father Burlando met another group of soldiers while on his way from Emmitsburg and was surprised when one of them called out, "Good morning, Father Burlando! How is Jennie Butts?" Jennie Butts was the Confederate soldier's younger sister, a Southern girl who was still in St. Joseph's Academy.[34]

While the Union Army had been on the grounds, Sister Mary Raphael Smith, the academy directress, and other sisters had had trouble making their girls from the Southern States act civilly toward the soldiers. One student wrote in a letter to a friend, "I am all in tremble afraid I will be caught. Last night we had a good *Lecture* about singing *political* songs we are forbidden to do it any longer we got the very mischiev for it every day we get a scholding…"[35] Political songs, in this case, meant Confederate songs.

Though the sisters had been polite to the Union Army, it is not too surprising that there were strong Southern sympathies on the campus. Most of the students left were girls from the Confederate States who hadn't been able to return to their families.

Once the Confederate Army appeared, the sisters became too enthusiastic. When the soldiers first approached, the girls set all rules and discipline at defiance and called out from the avenue,

James Rada, Jr.

"Give me a button! I'm from South Carolina!" Another shouted, "I'm from Louisiana."[36] Buttons were considered prized souvenirs for romantic young women.

Despite the warm welcome, the Confederates stayed only a short time before heading north themselves.

The following morning, the 107th Regiment, Pennsylvania Volunteers, Second Division First Corps marched through Emmitsburg on their way to Gettysburg. As they passed by St. Joseph's Academy, they were greeted by the sight of a long line of girls and Daughters of Charity along the side of the road.

At a word from the sister in charge, the females dropped to their knees and lifted their faces to the sky. They then began praying for the spiritual and physical safety of the soldiers marching to battle.

The scene touched the men who stopped, removed their caps and bowed their heads until the women had finished the prayer.[37]

The soldiers then continued their march.

Not long after, the calm of the day was shattered by the booming of distant cannon. Father Burlando wrote, "While the cannon's roar announced the vengeance of God on the iniquities of man, our Sisters were at prayer in the Chapel imploring mercy for all."[38]

The Battle of Gettysburg had begun.

CHAPTER 13
Gettysburg

"I do not know just when the devoted Sisters of Charity from Emmitsburg came to the aid of the wounded in the Catholic Church, but it was probably Saturday, the third of July, while the battle was still raging. Oh, how tender and welcome were their services to the poor suffering boys, to whom a gentle hand was everything in their wretchedness! They were constant in their work and devotion to the wounded."

Colonel H. S. Huidekoper
150th Pennsylvania Infantry

General Robert E. Lee had made his second incursion north through Maryland and then into Pennsylvania in 1863. His army met the Army of the Potomac under the command of Major General George Meade at Gettysburg in southcentral Pennsylvania. There on July 1, Lee's army came at the town from the north and west, pushing the Union out of Gettysburg to Cemetery Hill. In Emmitsburg, Sister Mary Louise Caulfield wrote:

Two hundred thousand men were in the field and on each side there were from one hundred to one hundred-thirty pieces of cannon. The roar of these agents of death and destruction was fearful in the extreme, and their smoke rising to heaven formed dense clouds as during a frightful tempest. The Army of the South was defeated and in their retreat left their dead and wounded on the battlefield.

James Rada, Jr.

What number of victims perished in this bloody engagement? No one yet knows, but it is estimated that the figures rise to 50,000. ... Our Sisters were at prayer in the Chapel imploring mercy for all.[1]

During the night, reinforcements arrived for both armies and on July 2, Lee tried to surround the Army of the Potomac. He first attacked on the Union's left flank at the Peach Orchard, Wheatfield, Devil's Den, Little Round Top and Big Round Top using Generals Longstreet and Hill's divisions. The next attacks were on the Union's right flank at Cemetery Hill and Culp Hill with General Ewell's division. The Union held Little Round Top and fought back most of Ewell's men.

On July 3, the Union drove the Confederates from Culp's Hill. Lee attacked the Union center at Cemetery Ridge and General Pickett charged the Union line. His men managed to pierce it but were pushed back and nearly decimated. General Stuart's cavalry attacked the Union from the rear but were repulsed.

That evening, rain fell and continued through the next day, leaving the ground soggy and muddy. While it made it difficult for the armies to move their supplies, it also hampered the efforts of those people who were trying to care for the wounded left behind on the battlefield.

On this last day of battle, Archbishop Francis P. Kenrick of Baltimore died. The archbishop had been Union in his sympathies but not necessarily anti-slavery. He believed that slavery under certain protective conditions was not in itself immoral, but he believed national loyalty had priority over state patriotism.[2] Reports were that his death had been hastened by his deep sorrow at the reports of the massive loss of life at Gettysburg.

Even as the Battle at Gettysburg was ending after three days, the months-long siege of Vicksburg was also winding down. Confederate General John Pemberton's 20,000-man garrison had shrunk through disease and starvation. City residents sought refuge from shelling in caves. Pemberton surrendered the city on

July 4. But General Ulysses Grant's victory in the South was somewhat overshadowed by a larger Union victory in Pennsylvania, which was much closer to civilians in the Union.

Lee began his withdrawal to Williamsport, Maryland, on July 3. His train of wounded soldiers stretched more than fourteen miles.[3] A few of the stragglers took a brief refuge with the sisters at St. Joseph's Academy before continuing South. Sister Camilla O'Keefe wrote, "On Sunday morning some poor straggling Confederates came down our way. ... They got a good warm breakfast here, after which they set out for part unknown to any but themselves."[4]

More than 50,000 men were killed, wounded or missing in the battle that engaged about 165,000 men. One of the dead was Union General John Reynolds. On the morning of July 1, he had been in command of the left wing of the Union army when the Confederate army approached along the Chambersburg Pike. He was supervising the placement of the 2nd Wisconsin in Herbst's Woods when he fell from his horse. He'd been shot in the neck and died almost instantly.

Reynolds' body was taken to Taneytown, Maryland, and then to his birthplace at Lancaster, Pennsylvania. On the day Lee began his retreat from Gettysburg, Reynolds was buried in Lancaster.

Reynolds' fiancée was a young woman named Catharine Mary (Kate) Hewitt from Oswego, New York. She and Reynolds had met when he had been commandant of West Point. Kate was a Catholic while Reynolds was a Protestant and much older than his fiancée. Still, they had fallen in love and planned to announce their engagement after the battle when Reynolds could get away on leave. As a promise, Reynolds had given Kate his West Point ring and she, in return gave him a medal and ring, inscribed "Fair Kate," that he wore on a chain around his neck.

They had also agreed that she would join a religious community if he were killed. Kate kept her promise to her beloved and entered the Daughters of Charity in March 1864. She received the name Sister Hildegarde and became a teacher. She eventually withdrew from the community in less than five years without making vows.[5]

After the heavy rains of the previous day had subsided, on Sunday, July 5, fourteen Daughters of Charity and Father Francis Burlando set out for Gettysburg in a carriage and omnibus, a journey of about nine miles. Because they had heard the sounds of the battle, they knew there would be wounded who needed care that they could provide. They had packed their carriage and omnibus with baskets of bandages, medicine and provisions.

The travel north was not without problems for Father Burlando and the sisters.

The Northern scouts were stationed here and there watching for the return of the Confederates. One of these bands seeing our carriage and omnibus and thinking that they were the ambulances of the enemy, were ready to fire on us. Later we reached a double blockade of zig-zag fence across the road. We wondered whether we dare go around it by turning into the fields, for in the distance we saw soldier, half hidden in the woods, watching us. Father Burlando tied his white handkerchief to his cane and holding it high, walked towards them while we also alighted and walked about so that they might see the cornettes. They viewed Father sharply, for they had resolved to refuse the Flag of Truce were it offered, but the cornette assured them that all was well.[6]

The soldiers lowered their weapons and moved the barrier across the road – a line of tree stumps – to the side to the carriage and omnibus could pass.

"As we passed, the pickets lifted their caps and bowed showing their pleasure on seeing the Sisters going up to attend the sufferers," Sister Matilda Coskery wrote.[7]

The small caravan came upon the battlefield suddenly and

they were shocked. Father Burlando wrote:

> What a frightful spectacle met our gaze! Houses burnt,
> dead bodies of both Armies strewn here and there, an
> immense number of slain horses, thousands of bayonets,
> sabres, wagons, wheels, projectiles of all dimensions,
> blankets, caps, clothing of every color covered the woods
> and fields. We were compelled to drive very cautiously to
> avoid passing over the dead. Our terrified horses drew
> back or darted forward reeling from one side to the other.
> The farther we advanced the more harrowing was the sce-
> ne; we could not restrain our tears.[8]

Sister Matilda wrote a more-heart-wrenching account.

> But on reaching the Battle grounds, awful! to see men ly-
> ing dead on the road some by the side of their horses. – O,
> it was beyond description – hundreds of both armies lying
> dead almost on the track that the driver had to be careful
> not to pass over the bodies – O! this picture of human be-
> ings slaughtered down by their fellow men in a cruel civil
> war was perfectly awful. The battlefield a very extensive
> space on either side of the road – the east was Meads (sic)
> stand the west Lonstreet's (sic) on both sides were men
> diging (sic) pits and putting the bodies down by the doz-
> ens. One newly made grave contained fifty bodies of
> Confederates. -- ...in another spot might be pointed out
> where the body of such a Genl lay until removed to an-
> other location – in this frightful condition we found the
> Battlegrounds of that fearful Battle of Gettysburg.[9]

The group also witnessed the bands of soldiers assigned to
digging the mass graves for the fallen. There seemed to be no
order to their work. Where the bodies lay, holes were dug to bury
the men. If bodies were numerous, large holes were dug for mass

James Rada, Jr.

graves. At Culp's Hill, the sisters saw sixty Confederate soldiers buried in one trench.

Confusion still reigned in the town of Gettysburg as well. One member of the group wrote:

> At last we reached the city of Gettysburg. Here a large portion of the Army was guarding the battlefield. All the avenues and environs of the city were encumbered with soldiers, horses, wagons, and artillery carts. The inhabitants were just emerging from the cellars to which they had fled for safety during the combat; terror was depicted on every countenance; all was confusion. Every house, every temple, the courthouse, the Protestant Seminary, the Catholic Church-all were filled with the wounded; and yet, there were thousands still stretched on the battlefield with scarcely any assistance, it being impossible to provide for all.[10]

The group moved slowly through the muddy streets and crowds of people. They stopped at McClellan's Hotel on the downtown square in the center of Gettysburg. The hotel not only had guest rooms but large common rooms that would soon be filled with the wounded from the battlefield.

> Our little band of Sisters was disposed of by sending two to each hospital as far as their number went. Our headquarters were the parlors of McClellan's Hotel which had been set aside exclusively for the Sisters' use. All of the churches were filled with the wounded; the Blessed Sacrament had been removed from the Catholic Church and even its sanctuary was filled with some of the worst cases, especially men whose limbs had been amputated. Because we had to make our way to the town at a snail's pace it was one o'clock in the afternoon before our real work began but after that the Sisters labored heroically and with-

158

out respite.[11]

The arrival of the sisters at St. Francis Xavier Catholic Church allowed the medical personnel there to assist hundreds of wounded soldiers. So many wounded were in the church that the sisters could barely pass between them. Indeed, every large building in Gettysburg had become a hospital, in all more than 113 of them.[12]

Father Burlando heard some confessions and then returned to Emmitsburg. The sisters returned to McClellan's Hotel late that evening. Father Burlando wrote later:

> After making our first round to the sick and wounded we returned to the Hotel and took some refreshment, then we were off again to our patients. The weather was warm and damp as is usually the case where a large quantity of gunpowder has been used. We did not see a woman that evening. The feminine element had either escaped to the country or remained hidden in the cellars. The next day the women appeared in their homes and looked like frightened ghosts, so terrified had they been during the fearful battle, and no wonder! The Sisters lay on the floor that night and needless to say they did not sleep very much. On the following day Mother Ann Simeon sent us beds, bed-covering, cooked ham, coffee, tea, and whatever she thought the Sisters actually needed. Sister Euphemia, the Assistant, had gone to attend to the Sisters in the Confederate Military Hospital, which, though it was a source of comfort to the poor Sisters in the South, increased the labor of Mother Ann Simeon. On the second day a reinforcement of Sisters from Baltimore came to our aid.[13]

Though Father Burlando had work to do in Emmitsburg, he continued to visit the sisters at Gettysburg. Returning home each night having seen the horrors left behind on the battlefield, Father Burlando was troubled by visions of what he had seen. Even as he sat down to write his superior in France three days after his first visit to the battlefield, he could hear cannon fire to the Southwest and where such sounds could be heard death was sure to follow. He wrote:

> My God when will you give peace to our unhappy country! We well merit these frightful chastisements, and they will not cease until we shall have been well humiliated. Aid us with your prayers, because the American does not pray; -- and yet, without prayer how shall we appease the anger of God?[14]

Father Burlando realized that more help would be needed, but finding it among the Daughters of Charity was difficult. Many sisters were working at other hospitals in other states and were needed just as much there as they were at Gettysburg.

He returned the following day with more sisters to give aid as well as beds and blankets for the sisters.

The additional help came from sisters who arrived from Baltimore and it was much-needed help. Of the 650 doctors with the Union Army, 544 of them went with the army in the pursuit of General Lee.[15]

As the Daughters of Charity went about their work, ambulances were provided to carry clothing, supplies, etc. to the wounded. Sister Camilla O'Keefe wrote, "Hundreds of poor fellows lay on the ground with only their blankets under them; they were delighted when they could secure a little straw brought from some neighboring farm by a friendly hand."[16]

One sister was seen using a teaspoon to give a drink to a dying man. It was slow work for a man who would soon die from his injuries, but she was able to bring him comfort in his final hours.

The Daughters of Charity would carry the horrible sights of

the battlefield with them. The ground appeared plowed by the shells of the battle. Though many of the bodies had been removed to hospitals, others still remained exposed to the elements. And even where there weren't bodies, there was evidence that they had been there – knapsacks, bayonet sheaths and weapons strewn around.

The Daughters of Charity searched for wounded daily. At one point, they saw a red flag on the battlefield that stood in the ground next to a sign that read: "1700 wounded down this way." The sisters diverted in that direction until they found the wounded. Mother Ann Simeon wrote:

> O, yes for some were in a frightful condition. The Sister too brought plenty of the vermin along on their clothes! – I shudder on thinking of this part of the Sisters sufferings. … The weather was very warm. We noticed one large man whose leg had to be taken off another part of his body was in such a condition that the big maggots were crawling on the ground on which they crept from the body. Many others almost as bad but the whole of them were crawling with *lice* so that the Sisters did a great deal for those poor fellows by getting *combs* to get their heads clear of the troublesome *animals*.[17]

In an unusual incident, two Daughters of Charity—Sister Mary Veronica Klimkiewicz and Sister Serena Klimkiewicz—were providing care to the wounded soldiers on the battlefield. Sister Veronica was working amid death and carnage when she was given a very pleasant surprise.

> Going over a field encampment we found the brother of one of our Sisters who was in a hospital in the town. He had been wounded in the chest and in the ankle. The kind officer allowed him to be removed to the hospital where is Sister was stationed. They had not seen each other for

James Rada, Jr.

nine years.[18]

The sisters' work in treating the wounded at Gettysburg lasted for weeks. Three sisters spent their time working at one field hospital until all of the wounded could be moved to regular hospitals in New York or Philadelphia where more Daughters of Charity usually wound up caring for them.

Though the sisters' primary goal was to help soldiers recover physically, the care also gave them a chance to break down barriers. "This section of the country knew nothing of the holiness of Catholicity but believed much that was untrue. We expected to encounter some difficulty on that score but to our surprise all who met us lauded our charity. Bitterness had lost its edge and modesty might blush at the welcome and heartfelt greetings that met us everywhere," Mother Ann Simeon wrote.[19]

In one instance an "elderly gentleman" came to Gettysburg shortly after the fighting ending looking for his son. While he knew his son had been in the fighting, he had no idea of whether his son survived. While the man was sitting on a bench outside of the McClellan's Hotel, a group of sisters arrived with clothing for the wounded.

"Good God! Can those sisters be the persons whose religion we always run down!" the man said.

The hotel owner William McClellan told him, "Yes, they are the very persons who are run down by those who know nothing of their charity."[20]

McClellan told the man that many people were having the same reaction and that "some of them fairly swore that they would never again believe anything wrong of persons who would do what the Sisters had been doing on the battlefield of Gettysburg."[21]

The success of the Daughters of Charity in caring for the wounded also earned them more respect from the doctors they worked with. Upon arrival at one hospital, the surgeon in charge took the sisters to meet the other female volunteers.

162

"Ladies, and you, men and nurses also, here are the Sisters of Charity who have come to serve our men. They will give all the directions here. You are only required to observe them," the surgeon told them.[22]

Amid the carnage, the Daughters of Charity who nursed soldiers at the hospital established in the Methodist church in Gettysburg actually found amusement when they went to the commissaries for clothing and other necessaries. The person in charge of the commissary would see their religious attire and say, "Sisters, I suppose you want them for the Catholic church hospital."

"No," the sisters would say, "We want them for the Methodist church hospital."[23]

While at Gettysburg, Dr. A. B. Stonelake came to the hotel where the sisters were staying and inquired if any of the sisters who had served at Point Lookout were in the area. One of the sisters was nearby and Dr. Stonelake walked over to meet her and Father Burlando. The doctor had worked with the Daughters of Charity in Hammond Hospital at Point Lookout. He had been so impressed by their service and humility that he had been baptized into the Catholic Church.

The doctor accompanied the sisters into the field to help care for the wounded. Sister Camilla O'Keefe wrote of him:

This good physician not only performed the duties of his profession but after he had set and bandaged shattered limbs, he worked like a common carpenter. From a farmhouse he obtained a saw, an axe, some stray board and some nails, and in a short time he had the men whom we found lying on the ground, raised on a kind of frame which made the poor sufferers feel that they were in beds.[24]

Most of the prisoners they were helping were from Georgia and Alabama and knew little of religion. They hadn't been baptized, which was fine, since many of them didn't even believe in Heaven or hell.[25] So Dr. Stonelake took the time to talk to the prisoners and testify to them of his own religious experiences.

Some of the soldiers listened and began to make connections, saying, "The Sisters are Catholics, and surely they must be right."[26]

Before long, fifty of the men, some of them Confederate officers, converted and were baptized. The wounded had been taken to the Catholic church in town and they recovered under pictures of the Stations of the Cross hanging around on the walls, and a very large painting of Saint Francis Xavier holding up a crucifix to show the benighted pagans the sign of our Redemption.

The men lay on the seats of the pews, under the pews, in every aisle; in the gallery and in the sanctuary there was hardly room to pass between them. Their own blood, the water used for bathing their wounds, all kinds of filth and stench added to their misery. The very air was vitiated by the odor of gangrenous wounds but there was never a complaint from these heroic men. A considerable number of them were dying from lockjaw, and this demanded much time for giving drinks and nourishment. [27]

With few surgeons available, for many men, their first medical treatment came from the kind words of the Daughters of Charity.

One sister found a tall Scotsman lying under a pew with only his head visible. He suffered from lockjaw, a bacterial infection of an open wound that attacks the nervous system and causes spasms in the jaw and facial muscles. He was close to dying. The lockjaw had spread to other areas of the body and threatened to stop his breathing. Because the Scotsman had never been baptized, the sister sat with him and talked of God and the church.

A crowd soon began to gather to listen.

The Scotsman was too ill to be moved and so he was baptized where he lay, shortly before his death.[28]

In another instance, a young cavalry officer saw one of these impromptu baptisms of a nearby soldier. The soldier asked the priest to baptism him and the priest obliged him.

The soldier awoke the next morning and asked a sister, "Will Jack die?"

The soldier was referring to his horse, which had been injured in the battle. The sister didn't realize this and answered, "No."

"Will I die?"

"I think so," the sister answered quietly.

The honest admission upset the soldier more than the pain from his wounds did. The sister tried to calm him, but his anxiety only grew more agitated. In particular, he worried over his fear of receiving judgment for his life and that he had no religion.

"My poor brother, did you not receive baptism yesterday?" the sister asked.

"Yes, but I should feel religion."

The sister spoke to him of God's love in a quiet and soothing voice. The man relaxed and then smiled as his soul found itself at ease.

"I do believe I have religion," he finally told the sister.

The earnest soldier was still at peace when he died.[29]

The sisters didn't convince everyone, though. Another young soldier chose not be baptized in the face of death. A surgeon told one of the Daughters of Charity that she should baptize the soldier anyway. However, the sister honored the soldier's wishes. She was there to serve and not to force her religion on anyone.

When the soldier's father arrived to visit his son, the sister told the father that his son didn't seem worried about not being baptized.

"Oh, no," the father said. "My Lou is a good boy. He volunteered in his country's service, fought her battles, dies for her and that will do."

"Surely you are baptized?" the sister asked.

"Yes, but my son does not need it."

So when the young soldier died, his father took his unbaptized body home for burial.[30]

Four Daughters of Charity were assigned to care for the wounded at Pennsylvania College,[31] which had been converted into a hospital housing 600 men. Some of the worst cases were sent here.

With a scarcity of surgeons, the sisters could only dress the wounds of the soldiers and try to ease their pain through their careful ministrations. "Every morning when they returned, eight or ten dead bodies lay at the entrance of the college awaiting interment."[32]

Amid this carnage, the sisters brought so many men to baptism that they lost count. "Very rarely did any one in danger refuse baptism when we could give the time for it, but to hear the men call piteously, 'Come to me when you have finished with his wounds,' obliged us to do violence to every other duty," one sister wrote.[33]

So many wounded were brought to the college that some of them had to be housed outdoors. In one instance, two young soldiers lay on a blanket with a little trench about two inches deep dug around them to direct the rain runoff so that they lay in the mud rather than a pool of water.

Another time, a sister heard a commotion among the patients in the college hospital wards. She saw a group of men with guns pointed at a man. With no one else stepping in to help, the sister walked over to the group and put her hand on the man who seemed about to be shot. She pushed back the door of the surgeon's room and led the man through it while holding out her other arm to prevent the armed men from following.

Without saying a word, the men lowered their weapons and left.

A doctor came over to her and said, "Sister, you have surprised me! I shall never, never forget what I have just witnessed.

I saw the men's anger and all the excitement, but I feared my presence would only increase it. I did not know what to do, when you came and made everything right."

"Well," said the sister, "what more did I do than anyone else would have done? You know they would be ashamed to resist a female."

"A female!" exclaimed the doctor, "All the women of Gettysburg could not effect what you have done. No, no one but a Sister of Charity could have done this. Truly, it would have been well, if a company of Sisters of Charity could have been in the War, for then it would not have continued for four years. The Sisters can do what they please. I shall never forget this scene."[34]

Another soldier refused a sister's kindnesses, possibly due to the bias and intolerance toward Catholics at the time. The sister persevered and the man finally began to respond to her kindness.

When the sister found out that the man was in danger of dying from his wounds, she broached the subject of baptism. He said he was too old to worry about baptism. After making no progress with him for two weeks, the sister removed the miraculous medal from her chaplet and slipped it under the soldier's pillow while he was sleeping.

"Blessed Mother, I can do no more for this man," the sister said to herself. "I leave him to you."

The next morning when the sister visited the man, he asked for a drink and then told her, "Sister, I do not want any breakfast today, but I want to be baptized."

She told him that he needed to feel sorrow for his sins.

"I have cried over them all night and also for my obstinacy towards your kindness. Will you please forgive me?" the man asked.

The sister easily forgave him. She had just baptized him when he died.[35]

Though the Daughters of Charity were happy to see the ranks of American Catholics growing, they did not prohibit or work against other religious representatives from baptizing soldiers.

One young man worried that he couldn't be immersed in the waters of baptism because he was crippled.

"Sister, it is very strange that no one says baptism is so necessary but you sisters," the man said.

A nearby Protestant minister heard the soldier and said, "Yes, young man, I say baptism is necessary and I am a minister. If you desire it, I will baptize you."

The soldier considered this and said, "Well, if you do it as Sister would, you may, but Sister, I want you to stay right here and see that he does it right."

The minister explained how he baptized people. The soldier asked the sister if that was the correct way and she nodded that it was, and so, the minister baptized the soldier.

The soldier asked the sister to remain with him as he died and he prayed until his last breath. His final words were, "O Lord, bless all the Sisters of Charity."[36]

In another instance, a soldier noticed a sister giving a medal to Catholic soldier.

"Sister, you gave something to that man a while ago and he must be easier for he has not groaned since. Please give me what you gave him," the soldier asked because he was suffering from his own pains.

The sister did and told the soldier about what the medal represented and a prayer he should say.

Later, the soldier told her, "I do not long to live except to help my parents; the doctor says I can be saved only by the amputation of my limb. I cannot bear this."

The sister talked to the doctor about the young soldier and was told that his only chance at life lay in amputating his limb. The doctor worried that it might already be too late to save the soldier's life if an infection or gangrene had set in.

The sister begged the soldier to submit to the operation for his own sake.

"Well, baptize me first, and then promise me that the doctors will not take the medal off my neck," the soldier said.

Worried that the soldier might die, the sister baptized the soldier and told him he could keep the medal. The soldier agreed to the operation but refused anesthetic during his operation. Instead he kept the medal where he could see it.

Despite the pain of the operation, he murmured only twice. He said, "O, my mother, my mother!"

The soldier survived the operation and while he was recovered, the sister sent someone to teach him about the Catholic church.

Once the soldier was able to move around, he would often point to the sister and say to anyone who would listen, "There is the Sister who saved my body and soul."[37]

After the battle at Gettysburg, Satterlee Hospital received many of the wounded, bringing the total number of patients at the hospital to a record number of 6,000. The wards were crowded and 300 tents had to be erected on the grounds to house all of the wounded. One sister wrote, "the hospital [was] filled in every hole and corner with those who have been wounded."[38]

Extra doctors and nurses were on duty, but many soldiers still died of their wounds. Among the staff at the hospital were forty-three Daughters of Charity.[39] This was the greatest number of sisters who would serve there at any one time.

Soldiers who arrived on July 7 had been wounded on the first day of the battle six days earlier and they told of other soldiers more-gravely wounded who were still on the battlefield because there was no way to remove them.

Besides victories at Gettysburg and Vicksburg, Union forces captured the last stronghold on the Mississippi River on July 9, and by December, the Union controlled all of Tennessee.

Just as the Union Army was beginning to see success on the war front, problems broke out on the home front. Though the federal government had instituted a draft to keep its army strong, men who didn't want to serve could pay $300 or obtain a substitute. Draft riots broke out in New York from July 13 to 16 because of the unfairness of the system. Rioters broke into buildings and lynched people. At one point during the riots, some participants threatened to set fire to St. Joseph's Military Hospital, but the Sisters of Charity of New York refused to leave their patients.[40] Regiments under General Meade finally had to be sent to New York to put a halt to the violence.

During July 1863, Sister Euphemia left Emmitsburg heading south once more. She traveled with one sister and six girls from St. Joseph's Academy. The girls came with her because it was believed that as the need for hospital beds at Gettysburg grew, the academy would become another hospital so Sister Euphemia offered to return the girls to their families in the South.

They traveled first to Baltimore where they stayed overnight at St. Mary's Asylum. Their luggage and their persons were searched by soldiers in the city before they could travel further on their journey. The officers overseeing the women who were searching the sisters passed through the room at one point and stopped.

The girls noticed that he observed Sister Euphemia very closely; finally, approaching her, he said in a very respectful manner: "Madam, your appearance seems to me sufficient passport for yourself and those under your charge. I regret this delay, but it was unavoidable. I will order your baggage also to be delivered at once, without search." The children felt convinced that it was the serene and peaceful expression on Sister Euphemia's face that compelled the officer to render valuable service.[41]

Their travails did not end once they left Baltimore. The group traveled in a boat flying a flag of truce. For two days and two nights, the sisters barely had room to sit because the boat was so crowded. One of the girls wrote:

> Sister Euphemia seemed to think that she was the only
> one not deserving of pity. Sometimes she made us all in

turn sit so as to lean our head against her; and when we got to the hotel, she gave countless practical manifestations of her kindness and her thoughtfulness of others. We were delayed a week at Annapolis and during this interval, Sister Euphemia, in her irresistible way, persuaded the girls to spend their time sewing for the poor.[42]

After the boat trip, the sisters boarded a train to Petersburg, Virginia. It, too, was crowded and they wound up in the last car of the train as it passed through a large marsh.

"This was providential; for we had gone only half way when a sudden explosion occurred. The engineer's head was blown off and several persons were seriously injured," one of the girls wrote.[43]

The last car was the only one that escaped damage.   Sister Euphemia took action and began moving from person to person giving aid where she could. She even baptized two of the passengers. One of Sister Euphemia's charges wrote:

The responsibility of the guardianship of six young girls, the inconveniences, and the alarming circumstances that beset us on this trip never caused Sister Euphemia even once to lose her sweet serenity, or did it disturb in the least, he habitual confidence in God. In these circumstances, as in all others of her life, she seemed to close her eyes and rest on the bosom of Divine Providence.[44]

When fall came, the Daughters of Charity in Corinth, Mississippi, were busy as Confederate wounded from Nashville, Tennessee, were sent to them. The soldiers had been wounded defending Fort Donelson from General Grant.

"The wounded were now arriving in large numbers, but so exhausted by the loss of blood, the jolting in rough wagons, and the exposure of the fearful night, that many were too far gone for relief," wrote William G. Stevenson, a Confederate doctor who was in Corinth at the time.[45]

About 5,000 wounded overwhelmed the city and its surgeons. Stevenson wrote that because of the need to save as many lives as possible, "A much larger proportion of amputations was performed than would have been necessary if the wounds could have received earlier attention. On account of exposure, many wounds were gangrenous when the patients reached the hospital."[46]

Delay would have meant death, but amputation did not much improve the odds. According to Stevenson, eighty percent of those who received amputations died anyway and deaths averaged fifty a day.[47]

The arrival of the sisters brought order to chaos, according to Stevenson. In a few hours, he said things appeared calmer and cleaner to him. As in other locations, the presence of the sisters seemed to remind the soldiers that they were civilized men and not wild savages.

One soldier who had broken his arm freely vented his pain and rage on the nearby doctors and male nurses in the colorful language that backwoodsmen prefer. When another soldier began doing the same when the sisters were near, the first soldier told him to be quiet.

"Have you no more manners than to swear in the presence of ladies?" the first soldier told his companion.[48]

Point Lookout was another place where the Daughters of Charity served that saw its numbers swell after the Battle of Gettysburg. Besides having wounded soldiers fill and overflow the hospital wards at Hammond hospital, Camp Hoffman opened on August 1 about a mile north of the hospital. The prison camp could hold 10,000 prisoners and was the largest prisoner-of-war camp for Confederate soldiers in the war. Before the war was over, more than 52,000 prisoners would enter the camp. The wharf where the Daughters of Charity received supplies for the hospital also became a disembarkation point for prisoners who were marched off to Camp Hoffman.[49]

The number of prisoners quickly swelled to 20,000 Confederate soldiers. A fourteen-foot-tall fence was constructed around the camp to contain the POWs. Because of overcrowding, the prisoners were only given tents to sleep in. The close quarters and poor conditions took their toll on the prisoners as they grew sick with disease, suffered from exposure or slowly starved.[50]

More than 4,000 of the prisoners or around eight percent would die during their incarceration. Camp Hoffman developed a reputation as the worst camp for Confederate prisoners of war, but the Maryland Department of Natural Resources notes that prisoner death rate was less than half of the death rate of Confederate soldiers in the field.[51]

After the arrival of Confederate prisoners, federal authorities ordered all female nurses to leave in October as a result of the Union Surgeon General's office General Order 351 by order of Secretary of War Edwin Stanton.

The order's purpose was intended to delineate the duties of medical staff and Dorothea Dix, who managed the civilian nurses. Instead, the order's unintended consequence was that it undercut Dix's authority. Nurses under her authority needed a "certificate of approval" from Dix and countersigned by the medical director of the facility where the nurse would serve.

Furthermore, the surgeon in charge made nursing assignments through the medical director to Dix. The senior medical officer was also in charge of the nurses when they were on duty. Surgeon General Hammond could appoint any nurse he so chose with or without a certificate.[52]

When the order arrived at Point Lookout, the Daughters of Charity there prepared to leave along with the other women who were serving as nurses there.

Before the sisters could leave, though, the surgeon in charge said, "Remain, sisters, until I hear from Washington for we cannot dispense with the services of the sisters."

James Rada, Jr.

He sent a telegram to Washington and was given this reply, "The Sisters of Charity are not included in our orders; they may serve all alike at the Point, prisoners and others, but all other ladies are to leave the place."[53]

This exemption did nothing to endear the sisters to Dix or the nurses under her direction. Abby Hopper, who was the chief nurse at Point Lookout, wrote:

> The presence of Protestant women, with ability to regard the need of the sick, and to sympathize with suffering humanity is a treasure beyond price. And here I must be allowed to contrast such with the cold intercourse of Catholic nurses, who are the machinery of an Institution and do not minister to the broken-down in spirit.[54]

Though the nurses who had to leave weren't happy, that event did show the value that doctors placed on the service of the Catholic sisters.

Rather than bemoan the fact that they now had more than ten times the number of patients to care for with less help, the Daughters of Charity saw it as a greater opportunity to spread the Gospel. "Then, truly there was a harvest of souls gathered to heaven for hundreds after hundreds were brought that seemed to have been sustained for the regenerating waters, dying as soon as these were applied."[55]

On November 19, President Lincoln visited Gettysburg for the dedication of the National Soldiers Cemetery there. Though he was not featured speaker, his short marks would be the ones remembered as "The Gettysburg Address."

By December, the Union military authorities had shut down the military hospital in St. Louis. The Daughters of Charity assigned there were sent to new places to continue their work, including military prisons.[56]

CHAPTER 14
1864

"I would any time rather see a Sister than a general, for it was a Sister who came to me when I was unable to help myself, in an old barn near Gettysburg, where I was. She dressed my wounds and gave me a drink and took care of me until I came here."

Union soldier
Satterlee Hospital

The year 1864 began on a sad note for the Daughters of Charity and all Catholics, especially for the Sisters of Charity of New York. John Hughes, Archbishop of New York, died at age 66 on January 5. Hughes had immigrated to America in 1817 with his family and was a graduate of Mount St. Mary's College in Emmitsburg. A staunch defender of Catholicism, Hughes had become a bishop in 1842 and archbishop in 1850.

President Lincoln had met with him in 1861 and had asked for Hughes' help in the Union cause. Archbishop Hughes had refused an official government appointment, but he had agreed to visit Europe on behalf of United States government. He visited Paris, Rome, and Dublin attempting to bolster support for the Union.

Hughes' health had been failing for a year, so his death came as no surprise. Eight bishops and more than 150 priests attended his funeral. His body was buried in the crypt of the old St. Patrick's Cathedral in New York City.

The Daughters of Charity suffered a more direct loss when

Sister Regina Smith died. The fifty-seven-year-old Daughter of Charity had diligently attended to her duties at Charity Hospital during her time there. She had continued sending sisters on missions of mercy around the state and region, and some of them had never returned. Seven Daughters of Charity working in New Orleans died between 1861 and 1863, and this does not include any sisters who Sister Regina sent from Charity Hospital to serve outside the state and died.

Not only sisters, but soldiers died, too. Though Sister Regina did not know them as well as her fellow sisters, their deaths had weighed on her from their sheer numbers. When they died, their beds were not empty long before another wounded body filled it.

As her health had failed since the beginning of the war, "She would often gather the remaining strength of her weak body to visit various Hospitals, fearing some of the Sisters might be in need of something; she would almost anticipate the expression of our wishes. Oh! how glad she would have been to mount the stairs of the Hospitals and administer relief to the sick; but this she was wholly unable to do."[1]

On January 18, 1864, Sister Regina attended an annual retreat with some of the other sisters in New Orleans. On the fifth day of the retreat, she went to confession, presided over an evening meditation with the sisters and finally left the chapel.

"I am obliged to retire. I can no longer support myself," she told the sisters.

She nearly collapsed into her bed with a fever. Concerned, the other sisters called in a doctor to check on Sister Regina the next morning. The doctor found nothing alarming, which brought relief to the sisters.

However, she did not improve. She prayed throughout the night as the other sisters watched over her.

Around 3 a.m. on the morning of January 24, she turned to the sister watching over her and said, "I have slept well."[2]

The sister arranged Sister Regina's pillows, and the ailing Daughter of Charity closed her eyes once more.

* * *

No one suspected that the last hour had come for our beloved Mother, and the Sister in attendance was taking a
thousand precautions to prevent any noise that would
awaken her good Mother. More than four hours had
passed before the truth flashed upon us. Approaching
nearer and examining her features we recognized the fact
that our model, our staff, our cherished Mother was no
more. How impossible to describe our grief and surprise![3]

Sister Euphemia sent the official word to the Central House
of Sister Regina's passing. As word spread that Sister Regina
Smith had died, letters and visitors arrived recalling the sister's
kindness and charity. Newspapers honored her passing with
praise of her life's work. Meanwhile, Sister Euphemia appointed
Sister Avellina McDermott to succeed Sister Regina at Charity
Hospital.[4]

A small journal was found in Sister Regina's room after her
death in which she had written her thoughts and feelings during
the retreat. Her final words showed her unwavering love for Jesus Christ and her fellow sisters. They also showed that she felt
she had not done enough and recommitted herself to good work.
Her closing thoughts could serve as a fitting epitaph for a humble
sister: "These, O amiable Savior, are the resolutions I lay at Thy
feet; reject me not in Thy wrath, but receive my poor soul in thy
mercy."[5]

She who had been the first to take the American Daughters of
Charity into war service did not live to see how fully those ac-
tions bore fruit with acceptance and respect for the Daughters of
Charity and the Catholic Church.

On February 5, the Council of St. Joseph's decided that the
sisters in New Orleans had been too long without seeing any of
the superiors. Mother Ann Simeon decided to travel to the city
and visit the sisters in the area.[6]

Mother Ann Simeon and nine younger sisters left Emmitsburg for New Orleans on February 11. Father Burlando and Sister Mary Raphael Smith traveled with them as far as New York. On February 1, the Daughters of Charity sailed from the New York harbor heading south.

Though it was an uneventful voyage, sea travel did not sit well with some of the sisters. The continuous rising and falling of the ship on the ocean waves and the unsteadiness of the deck under their feet caused some of the sisters to get seasick.

When the ship stopped at Havana, Cuba, Mother Ann Simeon and one of the sisters (who served as an interpreter) went to visit the sisters at Santa Isabel's College. They returned to the ship with a large basket of fruit for the sisters who had remained aboard.

The Daughters of Charity arrived in New Orleans on February 22 to find the city celebrating George Washington's birthday. They walked from the dock to the Hotel Dieu, which served as a hospital when needed, and found that the sisters in the city hadn't expected them.[7]

"We made a beautiful procession up Canal Street in our blue aprons and not extra nice-looking cornettes. Sister Sophie de la Chaise said when we landed that we were not far from Hotel Dieu and that we could easily walk there but indeed it was a long walk, and we had had no breakfast except a little black coffee,"[8] Mother Ann Simeon wrote.

While Mother Ann Simeon had gone from the North to the South to visit the Daughters of Charity in New Orleans, General Ulysses Grant, who had been successful in his Southern campaigns, traveled north to assume overall command of the Union army in March 1864.

In St. Louis, Sister Othelia Marshall, the procuratrix, set out on her own journey with three sisters heading for Alton, Illinois. Their destination was the military prison where Union Army officials had requested their help. The prison was the former Illinois State Penitentiary for Criminals that had closed before the war began only to be reopened in 1862 as a prison for Confederate prisoners of war.

Father Burlando sent a letter to the procuratrix who was serving at Gratiot State Prison Hospital. In response to the letter, four sisters, including Sister Matilda Coskery traveled to Alton Military Prison Hospital arriving on March 16.[9] Sister Matilda wrote:

> Before reaching the main entrance, we had to ascend a very rugged road, well protected by guards. We thought that they had never before seen the sisters from the manner in which they viewed us. Here a residence would have been provided for us, but we did not think it prudent to accept.[10]

The prison was intended to hold up to 1,750 prisoners, but when the sisters arrived, the population was nearly three times that amount. It held Confederate soldiers, treasonous Union citizens, and guerrillas.[11]

The Union and Confederate prisoners were kept separate everywhere except the prison where the Daughters of Charity served. While the guards might not have recognized the sisters, the patients in the hospital did. Sister Matilda wrote, "[W]e heard, 'Sisters!' reechoed in every direction, as some of them had previously known us at the hospital prison in St. Louis."[12]

Hot summers, cold winters, poor sanitation, and poor nutrition had taken its toll on the prison population. Unlike Camp Hoffman at Point Lookout, the Alton Military Prison had a higher-than-average mortality rate that the sisters hoped to reverse.[13] Sister Matilda wrote:

> It was said that they died here from six to ten a day. The place was too small for the number of inmates who were all more or less afflicted with disease; some were wounded, others a prey to despondency, typhoid fever, diarrhea, and the small pox; consequently, the atmosphere of the

prison was filled with the most noisome exhalation.[14]

The sisters visited the prisoner-patients twice a day. Besides helping provide care to the men in the hospital, the sisters found a room where "we were in danger of falling through the rotten floor at any moment." They used this room to prepare food and drinks for the patients.[15]

When smallpox had broken out in 1863, a quarantine hospital had been set up on an island in the Mississippi River. Any prisoner showing signs of smallpox was sent to the island, and 300 of them never returned. The sisters visited the sick and wounded twice a day and cooked for them. The Daughters of Charity also visited the Federal Guards' Hospital and the smallpox island to give comfort where they could.[16]

The sisters tended to the health needs of the men and soon began to see improvement in their general condition. They also visited the smallpox island once a week to care for the soldiers there.

Mother Ann Simeon returned to St. Joseph's Academy on March 24. Shortly after that, Sister Genevieve McDonough, the directress sent from Paris to Emmitsburg five years earlier died from a stone in her bladder. Sister Severina Brandel served as the directress until Sister Adelaide Voisin, the new directress, arrived from Paris.[17]

At the end of March, Father Burlando, Mother Ann Simeon, and Sister Beatrice Duffy left Emmitsburg for Boston and from there on to Liverpool, England. The travelers were going abroad to represent the Daughters of Charity of the United States at a major celebration in the native diocese of St. Vincent de Paul held in Dax, France.

On May 1, a house a mile from the Alton Military Prison was turned into a hospital under the stewardship of the Daughters of Charity. However, by July 1, the command in Alton changed, and the new colonel in charge did not want the sisters' help with the wounded.[18] However, he was only one of a few at the hospital who shared this opinion. One of the sisters wrote:

> We could no longer get what was necessary from the prison resources. New guards were likewise placed on duty, who refused to let us pass to the hospital. Some of the old ones happened to be looking on and saw the difficulty; they became indignant and stepping forward said, "These are not ladies or women, but Sisters of Charity!" They were permitted to go on without further trouble.[19]

On May 4, General Sherman and an army of 110,000 men left Chattanooga, Tennessee, on their march toward Atlanta, Georgia. Fighting continued elsewhere with General Grant's troops engaging Confederate forces in the Wilderness Campaign and an attack on Richmond. The tides of war had turned in favor of the Union.

Bishop Martin John Spalding of Louisville, Kentucky, was named Archbishop of Baltimore on May 6, and installed on July 31, 1864, more than a year after Archbishop Kenrick's death. Bishop John McCloskey was named Archbishop of New York also on May 6 and installed on August 21.

While no one was irreplaceable, it certainly seemed to soldiers that the Daughters of Charity were close to it. Their work was noticed not only for the good it brought the wounded soldiers but for the positive effect it had on non-Catholics toward the Church. On May 6, Father Mariano Maller, C.M., the former spiritual director for the Daughters of Charity, wrote to Mother Ann Simeon while he was in Paris, saying:

> Great blessings are in store for the Americans, -- I mean especially the Sisters. The general disposition is very favorable. They are generous and grateful to God, and these two qualities never fail to draw down from heaven the

James Rada, Jr.

choicest graces. If it be lawful to judge of the future by
the past, what cannot we hope for! How wonderful Providence has been to you, -- and how faithful the Sisters to
follow the inspirations of grace and correspond to the received favors! God had foreseen the woful war and in the
unsearchable depths of His Providence and justice, God
had decreed to permit it to come, but at the same time He
had prepared you for so solemn a duty as the one you had
to be called to perform. Nor do I think all is over, for
when peace shall be restored, -- and may it be very soon!
– the impression made on the public mind shall not wear
off so soon, and you works shall go on; the increase and
vocations shall be multiplied in proportion. How beautiful
a day comes down on you![20]

This changing of attitudes can be seen following the Battle of
Petersburg, which began in June 1864. Lt. Col. Daniel Shipman
Troy, 60th Alabama Regiment (Montgomery), was one of the
many Civil War veterans who relinquished anti-Catholic sentiments because of the Sisters devoted and impartial care and ministry to victims from both the North and South. Troy, an Episco-
palian and son of a Mason, encountered the Daughters of Charity
at Washington in Lincoln Hospital after the Battle of Petersburg.
Shipman wrote:

One of the first things that impressed me was that the
Sisters made no distinction whatever between the most
polished gentlemen and the greatest rapscallion in the lot;
the measure of their attention was solely the human
suffering to be relieved; and a miserable wretch in pain
was a person of more consequence to the Sisters than the
best of us when comparatively comfortable.[21]

By the end of May, Satterlee Hospital had almost 3,400 patients. Sister Mary Gonzaga Grace wrote, "Indeed, it is as if we

were in the midst of a little city. Everywhere we turn we meet crowds of the maimed, the lame and the blind, going through the corridors and years as best they can. The wards are quickly filling up with rows of beds in the centre, as new arrivals are coming in every day from the recent battles."[22]

As the wards filled with patients, the wards overflowed and patients were moved into tents on the grounds. The patients the sisters removed tended to have gangrenous wounds, and many of those removed eventually died from the gangrene.[23]

Yet, the Daughters of Charity had gained a reputation of being nearly heavenly healers. In one instance, a soldier had been poisoned in the face. He wouldn't see a doctor because he didn't think it would do any good. The sister told him she had a remedy that had worked for another sister who had been poisoned.

"A sister?" the soldier said, amazed.

"Yes."

"Why I didn't know that sisters every got anything like that."

The sister told the soldier that, of course, she and other Catholic sisters could get sick. They were human like everyone else.

"But I believe they are not for the boys often say they must be different from anyone else, or from other people, for they never get sick and they do for us what no other person would do. They are not afraid of the fever, smallpox or anything else," the soldier explained.[24]

Another time, a recovering patient returned from a visit to Philadelphia, drunk. He staggered off to bed, but when a sister came by to give him his medicine, he struck her. The other patients in the ward were so outraged that they attacked the man and might have killed him except that the sister pleaded for them to stop.

The drunken soldier was put in the guard house, as much for his own safety as for what he had done. The sister pleaded for the commander to release him.

The chief surgeon did so, but he let it be known that he was only doing so because of the sister. When the man sobered up, he begged the sister for forgiveness and gave up drinking.[25]

In June, the commander of the Alton Military Prison received a letter from Colonel William Hoffman, U.S. Commissary General of Prisoners. The colonel accused the Daughters of Charity of carrying information to and from the prisoners and declared that their services would no longer be used at the prison. General Joseph Copeland replied to Hoffman, telling him that the accusations against the sisters were unfounded.[26]

On June 7, the Republican Party met in Baltimore, Maryland and nominated President Lincoln for re-election with Andrew Johnson, a Tennessean, as his vice president. Besides being a supporter of Lincoln's, Johnson represented Lincoln's efforts to reunify the country. He was the only southern U.S. Senator who did not resign when the Confederate States seceded. Lincoln had also appointed him military governor of occupied Tennessee in 1862.

The Democrats would meet in Chicago at the end of August and nominate General George McClellan, Lincoln's former head of the Army of the Potomac, for President and George Pendleton of Ohio for vice president.

The hospital in Frederick was once again filled to overflowing in July 1864.

Lieutenant General Jubal Early crossed the Potomac River at Shepherdstown into Maryland with a corps of about 15,000 men on July 5 and 6. It was the first move in General Robert E. Lee's plan to relieve the Confederate Army of some of the pressure it was facing from the Union Army in Petersburg, Virginia. If General Early could launch an attack against Washington City, then the Union Army would need to redeploy to protect the capital city.

By July 9, Early's men had moved south of Frederick and were preparing to cross the Monocacy River. Union General Lew Wallace and his men were greatly outnumbered by more than two to one, but Wallace deployed them along the Monocacy to try and stop the Confederate Army. Though Wallace's defeat was nearly inevitable, he was able to delay Early long enough so that Washington's defenses could be shored up enough to withstand the Confederate attack.

The day's fighting left 2,200 men dead, wounded or missing with most of them being sent to Frederick for treatment.[27] Sister Matilda wrote:

It was truly heart-rending to see the mangled bodies of those poor creatures, many of whom were in their agony when brought to the hospital. Then great was our sorrow to see that their consciousness was not sufficient to permit us to offer them some words of consolation and to remind them to bear patiently their sufferings for the love of Him in whose presence they were soon to appear.[28]

On July 22, General Mason Braymen imprisoned William Henry Elder, Bishop of Natchez, Mississippi, for seventeen days. In October of 1863, Bishop Elder had refused to include a prayer at Mass for President Lincoln and for the success of the Union over the Confederacy. He was also accused of changing the words of a prayer that should have been prayed for Lincoln to one asking for God's help for Confederate President Jefferson Davis.

Braymen's arrest order called this a "violation of his duty as a citizen of the United States, and of evil example to them under his ecclesiastical authority, he well knowing and was instigating and promoting rebellion and armed hostility against the lawful order of the United States."[29]

Bishop Elder surrendered himself to military authorities, but he also wrote to Secretary of War Edwin Stanton on July 30 to present his defense:

As for my own word, I state distinctly and with full sense

of my sacred office, an my responsibility to God, that in altering the prayer after the passage of the Ordinance of Secession, my motive was not to instigate nor promote hostilities, nor the overthrow of any government, violently or peaceably, not to influence any one's conduct or sentiment with regard to the movement then going on.

I simply acquiesced in a state of things agreeable to the Ordinance, whether wisely or unwisely. There seemed to be a universal acceptance of it, even by those who had before opposed it.[30]

Braymen suspended the order until he could hear back from the War Department as to how to proceed. No action was taken on the matter in Washington, and it was allowed to drop.

Back in Alton, residents asked the Daughters of Charity to continue their care of the wounded even after Colonel Hoffman had accused the sisters of espionage. The sisters stayed and served. Sister Othelia Marshall and four other sisters started a general hospital called St. Joseph's in the former School of the Immaculate Conception.[31]

In August, the sisters found themselves working among both Union and Confederate sick and wounded. The Union soldiers were in Hammond Hospital, and the Confederate soldiers were prisoners at Camp Hoffman. However, the Daughters of Charity were the only females at the two sites.

On the morning of August 6, the some of the sisters at Point Lookout found themselves in a massive storm. One of the sisters wrote:

We were at meditation in our chapel about 5:00 a. m. when suddenly a noise like thunder surprised us. Upon looking out, we saw the air was darkened with whirling sand, lumber, bedsteads, beds, stove pipes, roofs of houses, etc., etc. A raging tornado and water spout was tearing and destroying all in its way, taking us in its course, from the river to the bay. Our poor little chapel shook from roof to foundation, doors and windows being blown down, and part of the walls giving way. Men, sick and wounded, were blown out on the ground, and the wards and cottages carried several feet from their base.[32]

Two sisters who had worked late were sleeping when the storm brought them awake suddenly because their room was being torn apart by the winds. Terrified, they ran outside. "In their efforts to reach the chapel they were struck down by the falling boards, etc., and as often raised from the earth by the violent wind,"[33] one of the sisters wrote.

Though scared, the Daughters of Charity sought to care for their religious symbols. One sister grabbed the tabernacle because she feared that it might be swept out into the bay.

Lumber and iron bed steads were carried over the tops of the cottages. The wards had been nearly full of patients, and several of these wards were leveled to the ground. The men who were able to move about were running in all directions for safety, many of them only half-dressed. The dead house was seen whirling through the air, and the bodies which were in it were not discovered for some time after the storm.[34]

The storm only lasted about fifteen minutes, but they had been fifteen minutes that showed the fierceness of Mother Nature. Once it abated, the sisters took the sacred liturgical vessels and sacramentals used in religious worship to an undamaged cottage. However, it took much longer for other buildings to be repaired. Meanwhile, the sisters still had patients who needed their care. "The sisters would stand by the stove with their saucepan of broth in one hand and an umbrella in the other, too happy that they were relieving the suffering men,"[35] one of the sisters wrote. Given the nearness of Camp Hoffman to Hammond Hospital, the Daughters of Charity also found themselves caring for the physical and spiritual needs of prisoners as well as Union soldiers. In one instance, the camp provost notified the sisters that a deserter was going to be shot in the morning and they might want to talk to him so he could make his peace with God. The sisters walked the half mile out to the camp, but upon arrival, the deserter would not see them. They returned to their quarters and prayed for the man's soul.

That evening, the provost sent an orderly to the sisters, saying that the deserter had had a change of heart and wished to speak with them. The sisters told the orderly that they could not go out walking in the woods in the dead of night.[36]

The orderly returned a short time later with a note from the provost that read, "I, on horseback will be your pilot to the ambulance I will send for you. I will show the driver safely through the little woods we must pass and I will conduct you home safely. I think circumstances require your corresponding with the desires he expressed, for they are very earnest."[37]

The sisters accepted the offer and were taken to the camp where they found a Protestant minister of the deserter's faith talking with the soldier. They waited for a couple of hours wondering if the minister had prepared the deserter for death.

When the minister left, the sisters were allowed to see the soldier. He thanked them for coming and apologized for having turned them away earlier. When the sisters found out that the young man had never been baptized, they explained its necessity to him. This led to other doctrinal discussions.

"Oh! Why have I not known you sooner!" the young man told them. "Well, if you can baptize me, do so, I beg you! Oh! Why did I not know you sooner?"[38]

The sisters baptized the man and told him that they would send for the local priest. The deserter asked if the priest could not be sent for now. The provost told them that the priest wouldn't be able to get to the prison before the execution was scheduled to take place.

The young man nodded his understanding. "I deserve death and freely pardon anyone who will take part in it. I know that I must die by the hand of one of my company, but whoever it may be I forgive him," the deserter said.[39]

The sisters left him sometime later with a promise that they would be praying at the altar for him before, during and after the execution.

As the provost made arrangements to return the sisters to the hospital, he told them, "May I have such help at my death, and die with such dispositions."[40]

At the dreaded hour, the sisters knelt before their humble altar most fervently imploring our Divine Saviour to receive the soul of their poor friend. They continued there long after the sound of the fatal fire had told them that his eternal destiny had been decided. The soldiers remarked that everyone on the Point was present at the execution, but the sisters who had retired to pray for the poor deserter.[41]

Admiral David Farragut took his ships south and made his way through the mined areas of Mobile Bay in August. His ships defeated the Confederate defenses and blockaded Mobile, Alabama.

Father Burlando traveled to that area in August as well. However, while visiting the missions in the Mississippi region, he contracted typhoid fever and could not return to Emmitsburg until late September. Once home, two sisters cared for him in the Vincentian House.[42]

The symptoms and recurrences of the disease would plague Father Burlando for the rest of his life.

The same month, the Council of St. Joseph's recalled the sisters from the U.S. Army General Hospital in Frederick.[43]

Such a decision did not mean the fighting was winding down. General William T. Sherman entered Atlanta on September 2. By

November, the Union Army would be on their way to Savannah, Georgia. Behind them, they left a path of destruction.

November brought with it the Presidential election of 1864. At Satterlee, Sister Mary Gonzaga Grace wrote that all patients who could travel were given furloughs, some as many as thirty days, to return to their homes and vote in the election. "Very few remain, and the North Corridor is closed for the present. The camps are vacated,"[44] Sister Mary Gonzaga wrote. The President wasn't taking any chances on whether he would get re-elected or not. He wanted to make sure that the military vote, which was very supportive of him, was fully represented in the election.

With the recent Union victories, Lincoln had little to worry about. He carried the wartime election with 212 electoral votes to McClellan's twenty-one.

In December, the soldiers began returning from the furloughs and by Christmas Day, the Council of St. Joseph's asked Sister Mary Gonzaga to devote her entire time and attention to Satterlee Hospital because of the volume of work there. They also asked Sister Philomena Myers to act in Sister Mary Gonzaga's place as sister servant and administrator at the St. Joseph's Asylum.[45]

It had been a busy year for the Daughters of Charity in the military hospitals. Nearly two dozen sisters had been sent away to perform their services saving thousands of lives.

CHAPTER 15
At War's End

"To members of this order I am personally indebted. When prostrate with camp fever, insensible for nearly three days, my life was entrusted in their care. Like guardian angels these Daughters of St. Vincent watched every symptom of the fever and by their skill and care I was soon able to return to my post of duty."

Father William Corby
Chaplain of Meagher's Irish Brigade

When the Union forces under Admiral David Farragut appeared poised to take Mobile, Alabama, in 1865, the Confederate forces sent their sick and wounded who could not be evacuated to City Hospital in Mobile. They knew the Daughters of Charity would care for them and they would be safe. The sisters took them in, and although the hospital was crowded, the sisters found room for the additional soldiers.[1]

In the north, Satterlee Hospital was hit with a smallpox outbreak. The smallpox patients were moved to other quarters to keep the disease from spreading and Sister Josephine Edelin, a Daughter of Charity who had previously survived a bout of smallpox, took care of all of them. At one point, she had forty-five patients to care for alone.[2] The doctors seldom visited out of fear of catching the disease themselves. The sister wrote:

When the weather permitted, I visited those poor fellows almost every day. Like little children at these times, they

expected some little treat of oranges, cakes, jellies, apples
or such things, which we always had for them; they often
said: 'It was the sisters that cured them and not the
Doctors for they believed they were afraid of taking the
disease; our patients appeared to think the sisters were not
like other human beings or they would not attend such
loathsome and contagious diseases which everyone
shunned.[3]

That same month, General William Sherman turned north-
ward from his destruction in Georgia. By February 18, he had
taken Charleston, South Carolina, and a month later he was in
Goldsboro, North Carolina.

In February, the U.S. Congress adopted the thirteenth
amendment to the U.S. Constitution that forbids slavery in any
state. It would be ratified on December 6 after twenty-seven
states approved it.

As the Union army approached Lynchburg, Virginia, the
Confederate authorities moved their sick to Richmond. The Surgeon General of the Confederate Army asked the ten Daughters
of Charity in Lynchburg to take charge of Stuart Hospital and
care for the ill in Richmond, which they agreed to do.[4]

Stuart Hospital had opened the year before and was named
for General J.E.B. Stuart who had died at the Battle of Yellow
Tavern in May 1864. "The hospital is improvised from the barracks of the City Battalion, and with very little alteration and
some renovation, a neat, airy and commodious retreat for the sick
and wounded has been secured. Surgeon S. Meredith is in
charge, with Surgeon C. W. P. Brock as his assistant. The hospital accommodations are sufficient for five or six hundred patients,"[5] the *Richmond Dispatch* reported when the hospital
opened.

Around the same time, a surgeon in charge of Stanton Military Hospital on I Street in northwest Washington who had asked
for the Daughters of Charity to aid him received his answer that

sisters would be sent. Sister Camilla O'Keefe left from Emmitsburg with six sisters headed to Washington on February 27.[6]

Once the sisters arrived to help, the hospital, which could accommodate 600 patients, opened up. It was located near Douglas General Hospital in a long, wooden barracks.[7] When other military hospitals closed in Washington, many patients were transferred to Stanton Hospital.[8]

On March 1, the Council of St. Joseph's sent an additional sister to Stanton Hospital. Then three weeks later, a sister was assigned to Lincoln Hospital, one to Satterlee Hospital, one more to Stanton Hospital and one to the Alton Military Hospital to visit the prisoners there.[9]

In St. Louis, the Daughters of Charity ran innocently afoul of the military authorities. A woman in St. Louis gave Sister Winifred Mallon a cooked turkey. What Sister Winifred didn't know was that a note for one of the prisoners had been hidden under one of the turkey's wings. The note was discovered when the turkey was carved, and the prison officers arrested Sister Winifred. Though quickly released, the incident brought a lot of negative public relations to the Daughters of Charity and Sister Winifred was forbidden to continue her work at the prison. She also refused to identify the woman who gave her the turkey, which did not aid Sister Winifred in her proclamation of innocence.[10]

President Lincoln was sworn in for his second term on March 4, 1865. He and most everyone else knew that the war was winding down and the two opposing sides would have to find a way to live together once again. His speech took on a conciliatory tone toward the Confederate States.

His closing thoughts of his inaugural address would have been something that the Daughters of Charity would have agreed wholeheartedly with. "With malice toward none, with charity for all, with firmness in the right as God gives us to see the right, let us strive on to finish the work we are in, to bind up the nation's wounds, to care for him who shall have borne the battle and for his widow and his orphan, to do all which may achieve and cherish a just and lasting peace among ourselves and with all nations."[11]

In Virginia, General Lee's army attacked General Grant's forces near Petersburg and at Five Forks. Grant resisted and pushed back. On April 2, Lee had to evacuate Petersburg and Richmond. With his army now almost encircled by the Union army, Lee met Grant at Appomattox Court House on April 9, 1865, and surrendered. It was an unconditional surrender, but Grant allowed Lee to keep his sword and horse as a sign of respect.

Other portions of the Confederate Army soon followed. General Joseph Johnson surrendered the Army of Tennessee at Raleigh, North Carolina, on April 26. This was the other major army for the Confederacy. Other smaller groups would continue to surrender throughout the year, and Confederate President Jefferson Davis was captured on May 10.

The news of General Lee's surrender eventually reached Richmond where it caused a lot of anxiety. Sister Juliana Chatard wrote:

Medical stores, commissary departments, and houses of merchandise were thrown open. Liquor flowed down the streets, that preventing its dangerous effects, some confusion might be spared. Stores became public property. The city trembled from the blowing up of the gunboats in the river that bound the city on the east.

Towards morning we thought it best to secure Mass early, for fear of what a few hours more might show forth. We were preparing for it, when suddenly a terrific explosion stunned, as it were, the power of thought. The noise of breaking windows in our hospital and neighboring dwellings added greatly to the alarm, as it seemed for the moment as an entire destruction. Fearing it might be the bursting of the first shells, the good chaplain thought it better to give the Holy Communion to the Sisters, and then consume the blessed hosts. Presently however, we learned that the Confederates had blown up their own supplies of powder, which were very near us. Then followed the explosion of all the government buildings. We passed that eventful day with as much composure as our trust in our good Lord enabled us to do, though from time to time, we were in evident danger of having our house with its helpless inmates all destroyed.

After the surrender; a Federal officer rode up to the door; told us we were safe, that property would be respected, that he would send a guard to protect the house.[12]

The Civil War had cost the Union 360,000 lives and the Confederacy 258,000 lives. Battle wounds had claimed 110,000 Union soldiers and 95,000 Confederate soldiers. Illness and disease had caused more casualties than battle injuries. It is estimated that for every 1,000 Union soldiers who fought in a battle, 112 were wounded and for every 1,000 Confederate troops in a battle, 150 were wounded. In a battle like Gettysburg, this means that 20,745 of the 51,000 casualties were injured and many received treatment from the Daughters of Charity.[13]

By the end of the war, nearly 700 Catholic sisters from different orders had nursed both Union and Confederate soldiers in military and local hospitals, on transport boats on the Atlantic coast and on the Mississippi, and at temporary military encampments. Even though these valiant women risked life and limb to serve the sick and wounded soldiers from both sides, through the years, their contributions have frequently been overlooked in printed histories and film accounts of the Civil War.

Though the war was over for all intents and purposes, there was still one last act to be played out. While President Lincoln watched a play at Ford's Theatre on April 14, John Wilkes Booth

James Rada, Jr.

shot him in the back of the head. At the same time, an attempt to kill Secretary of State William Seward at his home failed, and an assassin who intended to kill Vice President Andrew Johnson lost his courage.

With the end of the war and the release of sisters who had served in the military hospitals, members of the Council of St. Joseph's turned their attention toward requests for new institutions. They also continued to provide long-term care for veterans in existing hospitals throughout the country.

On July 25, Surgeon General Isaac Hayes wrote a letter to Sister Mary Gonzaga Grace discussing the closing of Satterlee Hospital. The Council of St. Joseph's reassigned many of the sisters from Satterlee Military Hospital to other missions two days later, and others on August 23.[14] Some of the Daughters of Charity at Satterlee Hospital remained until all of the patients were either discharged or moved to the U.S. Soldiers Home, located in Washington, D.C. When the sisters finally withdrew, ninety-one Daughters of Charity had been on duty there from June 9, 1862, to August 3, 1865.[15] The Daughters of Charity would eventually serve at the U.S. Soldiers Home providing nursing services there from 1902 to1980.

In August, the doctors at Point Lookout asked the sisters to remain until all the sick and wounded were released or moved. The sisters had spent three years there.[16] On leaving, one sister ended her story, summarizing what many of the Daughters of Charity who served in the war effort felt:

Thus you see, we had many, very many occasions of making the virtues and character of our religious better known where it had been until now, either a matter of indifference, or it had been hated, really hated. Without being able to detail evidences of having benefitted these poor men much, yet, with rare exceptions they venerated and respected our religion, and many believed that it was the only right one the only religion. Many died bearing with them saving fruits of this, their newly received faith.

Peace being declared, preparations were made for a general removal, but, Oh! How many went to their Eternal home, while picturing their tenderest wishes, their earthly homes, friends, etc.

The doctors desired the sisters to remain until all the sick and wounded had gone. This done, they too left the Point. This was August 1865. Our dear Valley with its many blessed boons was a most delightful contrast with our last three years.[17]

In response to a request from Stuart Military Hospital in Richmond, Virginia, the Council of St. Joseph's named seven sisters to help with the sick and injured.[18]

On September 20, Father Mariano Maller in Paris wrote to Sister Mary Gonzaga:

The view of the immense hospital reminded me at once of two things, one the very sad, the other very pleasing. It is sad to think of so vast a ground filled up with patients, victims of a horrid war. It is pleasing to see the daughters of St. Vincent from ward to ward, like consoling angels, pouring the balm of consolation into the saddened hearts of poor soldiers, thus separated from the affection of their own families. . . . But now . . . the dreadful scourge of war is over. [19]

Throughout the war, Daughters of Charity from St. Joseph's Central House had served the wounded from the North and South with equal attention, except when barred from doing so. At the request of Father Francis Burlando in 1866, Sisters who had served at the various hospitals during the war sent written accounts of their experiences to St. Joseph's Central House. In their accounts of nursing activities, the sisters recorded in detail the spiritual assistance they provided for those under their care and listed many conversions, baptisms at death, returns of careless Catholics; they consoled dying or wounded patients and encouraged them to pray. Peace allowed the sisters to return either to their former mission and ministries or to new assignments, but their efforts were not lost on the patients under their care. Many veterans relinquished their anti-Catholic sentiments because of the sisters' devoted care.

Though the war had ended, the mission of the Daughters of Charity hadn't. In 1865, ninety-seven young women entered the sisterhood, which was a record number at that time. During the war, even when the Daughters of Charity's resources had been stretched thin, 477 women had entered the order, and nineteen missions were opened.

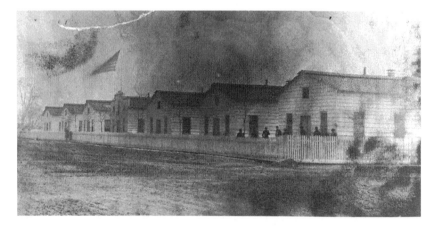

Stanton Hospital in Washington D.C. during the Civil War. Courtesy of the Library of Congress.

CHAPTER 16
The Admiration of Angels

"The war has brought out one result – it has shown that numbers of the weaker sex, though born to wealth and luxury, are ready to renounce every comfort and brave every hardship, that they may minister to the suffering, tend the wounding in their agony, and soothe last struggles of the dying. God bless the Sisters of Charity in their heroic mission! I had almost said their heroic martyrdom! And I might have said it, for I do think that in walking those long lines of sick beds, in giving themselves to all the ghastly duties of the hospital, they were doing a harder task than was allotted to many who mounted the scaffold or dared the stake."

Rev. George W. Pepper
U.S. Army Chaplain

The following is a letter that Father Francis Burlando wrote to Father Jean-Baptiste Etienne, C.M., superior general of the Congregation of the Mission and the Daughters of Charity, on April 10, 1865. The letter accompanied Father Burlando's notes about the services that the Daughters of Charity provided during the Civil War:[1]

Most Honored Father,
Your blessing if you please!
I have the honor to address you on the subject of your

199

good American Daughters in the course of this unhappy four years' war which has left so many ruins and caused such ravages, notably in the Southern part of our immense Republic.

These observations are very incomplete; all is not told. Facts most interesting and edifying have been omitted, either designedly and through prudence, or because God has not manifested to us in its whole extent the good which is His mercy, He has willed that your Daughters should be instrumental in effecting. What has been recorded, however, suffices for a general appreciation well calculated, it appears to me, to impress us with the grandeur of our vocation of Charity.

It was a spectacle worthy the admiration of angels and of men, two hundred and twenty Sisters of Charity multiplying themselves as if by a miracle in the North and in the South to respond to the needs of so many unfortunate persons. Some Military Hospitals counted as high as four thousand beds, occupied by poor soldiers whose mutilated and broken members presented a heartrending scene. Whence could the Sisters draw sufficient charity with the spirit of sacrifice to save from death these thousands of victims?

They would do so by their tears and by words which penetrate hearts and enlighten minds. For, from the first, our Sisters knew how to inspire patience, whilst infusing the balm of hope into stricken souls. Men whom the horrors of war had, as it were, deprived of all feeling were touched by the sight of a Sister of Charity in the performance of her duty. The remembrance of a mother, a wife, a sister was present to their mind with all the charm of virtue, and from their eyes, which the atrocities of war seemed to have forever dried, flowed again tears of tenderness. Nobler sentiments, principles of honor, and of generosity which distinguish man from brute, reappeared;

whilst the dignity of human nature in its resemblance to its Creator, could once more be recognized. They thanked God for having sent to relieve them in their distress, those whom they considered Angels, and the evinced only respect, even veneration towards these benefactresses whom they honored with the more entire confidence.

In the presence of the Sister not an oath, no free words, not even a disorderly sound. You would have taken these halls where lay several hundreds of wounded men, for so many cloisters inhabited by religious. Nothing was heard save sighs wrung by the violence of pain from the weakness of nature.

To respect and confidence was joined the docility of a child towards its mother. It was beautiful to see the General, like the simple soldier, transform himself into a little child.

Behold, to the honor of our holy Religion, how the prejudices of an education opposed to Catholicity were dispelled, extinguishing the implacable hatred which heresy had vowed, so to speak, from the very cradle. Protestants ask themselves with astonishment, and in admiration, if these women are really Catholics; some among them do not believe it possible that persons so charitable could belong to a sect so monstrous as the Papist. Thus do they express themselves in the presence of the Sisters. Meanwhile, not being able to understand the prodigy of a bad tree—such as they judged Catholicity to be—producing such good fruits through the works of the Sisters of Saint Vincent de Paul, they wish to know in what this religion consists. They devour the books which are lent to them; they investigate, inquire, and at last find what, in the sincerity of their soul they seek; they embrace this divine religion of which they had never heard except in terms that had led them to detest it. Others, however, not believing their own eyes, would wish to belong only

201

to the religion of these true Daughters of Charity, instead of to the Catholic religion.

The Sisters endeavored to enlighten them, and with such success that more than once in order to calm the anxiety of the dying, they were obliged with their own hands to administer the Sacrament of Baptism; only thus could they be convinced that they died veritably in the Church of God.

But what a spectacle to see these poor invalid Catholics and Protestants all going to the Sisters' chapel to assist at the Holy Sacrifice of the Mass, at the Way of the Cross, and other practices of piety. Those who could not come by the aid of crutches, wished to be carried there. What eagerness they manifested to obtain a medal of our Immaculate Mother, a Rosary, an Agnus Dei; and only after they had received a medal would they return satisfied to their regiments. In a word, one would have thought that a most fervent spiritual retreat was being kept in our hospitals by these brave soldiers resolved to save their souls. Thus were the merciful designs of Providence accomplished.

The great and the lowly could perceive the true light,--light reflected by the brilliancy of deeds of charity. Public authorities made it an obligation to proclaim aloud the exalted virtues and services of your Daughters. Many amongst them, instant in their praises, braved all prejudice at the risk of sacrificing position. A celebrated General went so far as to say that the Government and the American Nation were powerless to recompense them according to their merits. The nation had not remained insensible to this testimony. For the first time, Congress has decided to grant an appropriation to a Catholic establishment, by giving thirty thousand dollars towards the construction of Providence Hospital in Washington; undoubtedly not inasmuch as the work is Catholic, but because it is confided to the Sisters of Charity. Light will gradually dissipate the clouds which still obscure the truth, or veil the brightness of the full day.

The influence of the Sisters extended to both belligerent factions. The two Presidents seconded alike this policy of charity which occupied itself in ministering to the body, whilst having only in view the salvation of the soul.

I should not omit to mention, Most Honored Father, and for the greater glory of God, that your Daughters had shown themselves faithful to their practices of piety, even amid a thousand embarrassments arising from the trouble, disorder, and confusion, which, notwithstanding the firmest discipline, war inevitably brings in its train; above all, under the influence of conflicts incessantly renewed, and forever threatening.

After great battles the wounded were brought in, covered with dust and blood, by hundreds and thousands and the greater portion half dead. Under such circumstances how could it be possible not to sacrifice oneself utterly for the solace of such misery? The Sisters have barely time to take their repasts, and at night a few moments repose.

Now, we must consider the subject of the Sisters and their great, limitless Rule. Outside of duty, there was fidelity to the Rule in its entirety. Exercises were performed at the hour indicated, as if by the clock of the Community, and none would at such times dare to disturb the Sister in the accomplishment of her religious duties. Catholics and Protestants had faith in the efficacy of prayer, and they themselves became recollected in seeing the Sisters pray.

In was from prayer, indeed, that our Sisters drew the courage, the strength, and the graces which were so necessary in the midst of their many trials. Most certainly in instructing them how to acquit themselves with success of their duty, it was not forgotten at the Central House to prepare them for their mission, and by salutary advice to forewarn them against the dangers to which they would incessantly be exposed; but it must be admitted that by the grace of God, their exactitude to conform to these wise counsels merits to be proposed as a model worthy of imitation. In the visits which I deemed it of obligation to make, I had the consolation of hearing these edifying words: "Father, here we follow all our exercises of piety: Mass, Communion, Spiritual Reading, the Chaplet, even the observance of silence as at the Central House. My companions are full of fervor and zeal. I assure you that it is not impossible to live here, with just the same regularity as in a cloister."

Remarkable words, which render more sacred to us even in their slightest prescriptions, the deposit of our Holy Rules. Therefore, I am led to insert these words in this correspondence, assured that the Sisters who have put them in practice before uttering them, will have sufficient humility by the grace of God to preserve their fruits.

Most Honored Father, God could not withhold His blessing from labors undertaken in such a spirit. Called for the first time, to exercise their services on the battlefield, our Sisters were without practical experience; for this reason I was slow to acquiesce to the desires and solicitations of many who urged me to offer to the Government the assistance of the Sisters for the work of the ambulances. It was to be feared, moreover, that even were they apt at this kind of service, might they not stray from the spirit of regularity which seems incompatible with camp life? However, the Divine Will was manifest through the medium of Superiors, and I cast aside these fears to count more assuredly upon the succor of Almighty God, as we were conforming to the designs of His Providence. Truly, our Sisters, to the number of two hun-

dred and twenty, dispersed over North and South, upon
the fields of battle, under the floating tents of ambulances,
and within the walls of hospitals, have been the instruments of salvation which the grace of vocation has
wrought everywhere. It was admirable to see young Sisters hitherto engaged only in the work of schools, become
all at once, expert nurses, guided certainly, but a super-
natural instinct in their ministrations of the sick.

The Doctors could not repress their astonishment. Not
a regret to admit, Most Honored Father, but on the contrary, felicitations without number to gather; eternal gratitude from the thousands of victims who have been suc-
cored, saved from the death of the soul, as often as from
that of the body.

Such is the triumph which Heaven prepares for the
Catholic religion in the minds and hearts of Protestant
populations. What prejudices dissolved, what virtues in-
spired! How many souls rescued,--God alone knows the
number! Now, may we not believe that our holy Religion
has germs of life planted at every point of this vast Republic? Soldiers restored to health, in whose hearts the
benefits of charity have cast these needs, are to be found
in all parts. How could it be otherwise than that this sign
of charity should have known the true Religion? It is the
promise of Our Savior in all its Splendor: "By this shall
all men know that you are my disciples, if you have love
one for another." Again, the Sister of Charity is as much
at home in these immense regions, which she can traverse
from one extremity to the other—from Boston to San
Francisco—as in the bosom of her family, having nothing
to fear, assured of the triumph which gratitude has secured to her in hearts. The soldiers attended by the Sisters
of Charity make it their glory to proclaim the material
care which they have received from them. These monu-
ments must be more lasting, as we trust, than those of

James Rada, Jr.

marble and bronze; they express more forcibly the regenerating power of Catholicity upon souls. It is difficult to
resist arguments of this kind; they impose silence on
calumny, and cause to be respected by its enemies, a religion which they admire, and of which the Pope, whom
they do not recognize as yet, is nevertheless, the Supreme
Pastor. To insult the Roman Pontiff, after benefits through
which they have been made objects of predilection on the
part of his sheepfold, would be to cover themselves with
confusion, and expose themselves to the malediction of
the whole world.

It is to these miracles of charity, Most Honored Father, rather than to the wonders wrought by adepts in
physical science that may be attributed the light of truth
which now begins to illuminate, more than ever, our
America after the bloody catastrophes, the disasters, and
the chaos of our deplorable Civil War. May God be eter-
nally blessed, moreover, for the era of happiness which is
in His mercy, He opens before us, after the overwhelming
manifestation of His justice!

Your devoted son in Christ Jesus,
F. Burlando, C.M.

Many of the soldiers who received care from the Daughters
of Charity during the Civil War never forgot their battlefield angels or the care the sisters gave them.

After the war, Sister Mary Conlon's remains were exhumed
from Point Lookout where she had died of typhoid fever and tak-
en to Washington City for reburial in Calvary Cemetery. The
soldiers who assisted with the exhumation and reburial showed
the remains a great reverence while they handled them.

On December 13, 1862, Union soldiers had attacked the Confederate stronghold called Marye's Heights. Thomas Trahey of
the Sixteenth Michigan Volunteers was wounded in the fighting

and taken to an emergency hospital. There Sister Mary Louise La Croix cared for him until he was well enough to be sent home.

After the war, Trahey wrote to the Central House asking after Sister Louise. He was told that she had died two years after the war had ended and was buried in St. Louis. Trahey located her grave and began making an annual pilgrimage there.

On October 15, 1874, Catholic Sisters Josephine Meagher and Rachel Conway, were chosen to unveil a monument at former President Abraham Lincoln's tomb in Oak Ridge Cemetery in Springfield, Illinois. The memorial recognized the service of the Catholic sisters in the war.

On September 20, 1924, a marble and brass memorial called "The Nuns of the Battlefield" was dedicated in Washington D.C. to all of the religious orders that provided nurses during the Civil War. The monument is located at the intersection of Rhode Island Avenue NW and M Street NW opposite of St. Matthew's Cathedral. The Ladies' Auxiliary of the Ancient Order of the Hibernians paid for the monument.

At the time of the dedication, only three Catholic sisters were still alive who had given wartime service during the Civil War. Sister Mary Madeline O'Connor, an 81-year-old Catholic sister. "Made brilliant by the robes of the high officials of the church and the uniforms of soldiers, sailors, and marines, the dedicatory services attended by upward of 5,000 persons, were impressive,"[2] reported the *Sandusky Star-Journal*.

Archbishop William Cardinal O'Connell told the audience:

Should the time ever come that this nation faced the horrors of war… Then, too, will come out of their cloistered homes another band of ministering angels, the spiritual heirs of holy nuns, whose sacred memory we here venerate, and they, like those here honored, will bring to the fallen aid and consolation, courage and resignation.[3]

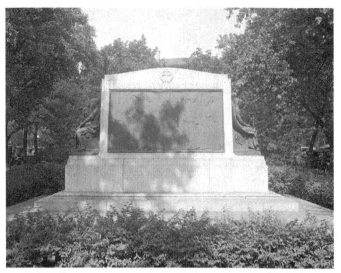

The Nuns of the Battlefield Memorial in Washington D.C.
(above) Archbishop O'Connell at the dedication of the Nuns of
the Battlefield Memorial (below). Courtesy of the Library of
Congress.

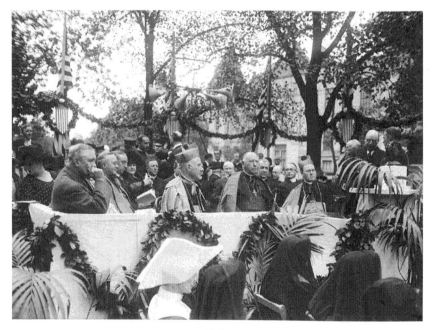

APPENDICES

APPENDIX A

Cities and Military Hospitals Where the Daughters of Charity Served in the Civil War [1]

The Daughters of Charity cared for military patients from both the Union and Confederate armies in military hospitals and hospitals operated by the Daughters of Charity at these locations.

City	Years	Type	# of DOC	Patients
ALABAMA				
Mobile	1862	City Hospital	unk.	CSA
		Marine Hospital	7	CSA
Montgomery	1861	unk.	unk.	Both
DISTRICT OF COLUMBIA				
Washington	1862-65	Providence Hospital	unk.	Union
		Eckington Hospital	unk.	Union
		Cliffburne Hospital	unk.	Union
		Lincoln Hospital	unk.	Union
FLORIDA				
Warrington	1861	Improvised	6	CSA
GEORGIA				
Atlanta	1863	Tents	5	CSA
Marietta	1863	Hospital	5	CSA
ILLINOIS				
Alton	1862-65	Military Prison	4	Both
LOUISIANA				
Camp Moore	1861	Camp Hospital	4	CSA
Monroe	1862-63	Camp Hospital	3	CSA
New Orleans	1861-62	Charity Hospital	unk.	CSA
		Hotel Dieu	unk.	Union
		Marine Hospital	unk.	CSA
MARYLAND				
Antietam	1862	Fields - Improvised	2	Both
Boonsboro	1862	Fields - Improvised	2	Both
Frederick	1862-64	Hessian Barracks	10	Both
Point Lookout	1862-65	Tents	26	Both

Sharpsburg	1862	Improvised	2	Both
MISSISSIPPI				
Holly Springs	1861-62	Temporary Hospital	4	CSA
Natchez	1862-63	Unk.	3	CSA
MISSOURI				
St. Louis	1862	2 Military Prisons	3	Both
PENNSYLVANIA				
Gettysburg	1863	Many Improvised	Unk.	Both
Philadelphia	1862-65	Satterlee &		
		St. Joseph's Hosp.	43	Both
VIRGINIA				
Danville	1862	Improvised	10	CSA
Gordonsville	1862	Military Hospital	3	CSA
Lynchburg	1862-65	Factory Hospital	5	CSA
Manassas	1862	Improvised	5	Both
Norfolk	1861	St. Vincent's Hospital	5	CSA
Portsmouth	1861	Marine Hospital	Unk.	Union
Richmond	1861-65	St. Francis de Sales	Unk.	CSA
		General Hospital	Unk.	Both
		Others	Unk.	CSA
White House Sta.	1862	Improvised and Ships	130	Union
Winchester	1861	Hospital	6	CSA
WEST VIRGINIA				
Harpers Ferry	1861	Hospital	3	Both

APPENDIX B

Civil War Battles Where the Daughters of Charity Served[2]

Though the Daughters of Charity served in many capacities, the most-dangerous location was on the battlefields. The following are some of the major battles where the sisters were actually on the battlefield. The casualty numbers are the estimated killed, wounded and missing from the campaign.

Conf. Force	Casualties (%of force)	Union Force	Casualties (%of force)	Total Cas.
GETTYSBURG *(July 1-3, 1863)*				
75,000	28,063 (37%)	83,000	23,049 (28%)	51,112
7 DAYS BATTLE (June 25-July 1, 1862)				
95,000	20,614 (22%)	91,000	15,849 (17%)	36,463
ANTIETAM (September 17, 1862)				
52,000	13,724 (26%)	75,000	12,410 (17%)	26,134
2nd MANASSAS (August 28, 1862)				
49,000	9,197 (19%)	76,000	16,054 (21%)	25,251
1st MANASSAS (July 21, 1861)				
32,230	1,750 (5%)	28,450	2,950 (10%)	4,700
SOUTH MOUNTAIN (September 14, 1862)				
18,000	2,685 (15%)	28,000	1,813 (6%)	4,498
WINCHESTER/BOWERS HILL (May 25, 1862)				
16,000	400 (3%)	6,500	2,019 (31%)	2,419

James Rada, Jr.

APPENDIX C

Orders of Catholic Sisters Who Served and Their Numbers[3]

Order	Sisters Served	Percent of Total
Daughters of Charity (Emmitsburg, MD)	300	43.2
Sisters of the Holy Cross (Notre Dame, IN)	63	9.1
Sisters of Charity of Cincinnati (Cincinnati, OH)	38	5.5
Sisters of Charity of Kentucky (Nazareth, KY)	37	5.5
Sisters of Mercy (Pittsburgh, PA)	34	4.9
Sisters of Saint Dominic (Springfield, KY)	24	3.5
Sisters of Mercy (Baltimore, MD)	22	3.2
Sisters of Mercy (Vicksburg, MS)	18	2.6
Sisters of Our Lady of Mercy (Charleston, SC)	18	2.6
Sisters of Saint Dominic (Memphis, TN)	16	2.3
Sisters of Mercy (New York, NY)	15	2.2
Sisters of St. Joseph (Philadelphia, PA)	14	2.0
Sisters of Charity of New York City (New York, NY)	13	1.9
Sisters of Mercy (Cincinnati, OH)	11	1.6
Sisters of Providence (St. Mary of the Woods, IN)	11	1.6
Sisters of the Poor of Saint Francis (Cincinnati, OH)	10	1.4
Sisters of St. Joseph (Wheeling, WV)	10	1.4
Sisters of Mercy (Chicago, IL)	10	1.4
Sisters of Our Lady of Mt. Carmel (New Orleans, LA)	9	1.3
Sisters of Mercy (Little Rock, AK)	8	1.2
Sisters of Saint Dominic (Springfield, IL)	6	0.9
Sisters of Saint Ursuline (Galveston, TX)	6	0.9
	693	100.2*

* Totals to more than 100 percent due to rounding.

212

About the Author

James Rada has written many works of historical fiction and non-fiction history. They include the popular books *Saving Shallmar: Christmas Spirit in a Coal Town, Canawlers,* and *Secrets of Garrett County.*

He lives in Gettysburg, Pa., where he works as a freelance writer. James has received numerous awards from the Maryland-Delaware-DC Press Association, Associated Press, Maryland State Teachers Association, Society of Professional Journalists, and Community Newspapers Holdings, Inc. for his newspaper writing.

If you would like to be kept up to date on new books being published by James or ask him questions, he can be reached by e-mail at jimrada@yahoo.com.

To see James' other books or to order copies on-line, go to www.jamesrada.com.

PLEASE LEAVE A REVIEW
If you enjoyed this book, please help other readers find it. Reviews help the author get more exposure for his books. Please take a few minutes to review this book at Amazon.com or Goodreads.com. Thank you, and if you sign up for my mailing list at jamesrada.com, you can get FREE ebooks.

Endnotes

CHAPTER 1

[1] Daughters of Charity, *Mother Regina Smith and Mother Ann Simeon* (Emmitsburg, MD: St. Joseph's, 1939) p. 60.

[2] Sister Daniel Hannefin, *Daughters of the Church: A Popular History of the Daughters of Charity in the United States 1809-1987* (Brooklyn, NY: New City Press, 1989) p. 130.

[3] Hannefin, p. 53.

[4] Frank R. Freemon, *Gangrene and Glory: Medical Care During the American Civil War* (Urbana, IL: University of Illinois Press, 2001) p. 28.

[5] Daughters of Charity. Act of Incorporation. Archives of St. Joseph's Provincial House (ASJPH) Emmitsburg, MD. January 1817.

[6] *Mother Regina*, p. 59.

[7] Hannefin, p. 130.

[8] Hannefin, p. 131.

[9] *Mother Regina*, p. 1.

[10] *Mother Regina*, p. 1.

[11] *Mother Regina*, p. 3.

[12] Sister Mary Bernard McEntee, D.C. *The Valley* (Emmitsburg, MD: Saint Joseph College Alumnae Association, 1972) p. 9.

[13] McEntee, p. 11.

[14] ASJPH 3-3-5-1821:60.

[15] *Mother Regina*, p. 3.

[16] *Mother Regina*, p. 4.

[17] *Mother Regina*, p. 4.

[18] *Mother Regina*, p. 10.

[19] *Mother Regina*, pp. 18-19.

[20] Hannefin, p. 53.

[21] Hannefin, pp. 53-54.

[22] Hannefin, p. 54.

[23] Chaves-Carballo E. "Carlos Finlay and yellow fever: triumph over adversity," *Military Medicine,* October 2005, 170: 881–5.

[24] John E. Salvaggio, *New Orleans' Charity Hospital: A story of physicians, politics and poverty* (Baton Rouge, LA: LSU Press, 1992) p. 47.

[25] Hannefin, p. 54.

[26] Hannefin, p. 55.

[27] *Mother Regina*, p. 36.

[28] *Mother Regina*, p. 58.

CHAPTER 2

[43] Jefferson Davis's Inaugural Address, Montgomery, Alabama, February, 1861, *www.civilwarhome.com/davisinauguraladdress.htm*

[44] Abraham Lincoln First Inaugural Address, Monday, March 4, 1861, *www.bartleby.com/124/pres31.html*

[45] Vincent de Paul; 10:507, as quoted in Pierre Coste, C.M., *The Life and Works of Saint Vincent de Paul*, tr. By Joseph Leonard (Westminster, 1952), 2:438.

[46] *Times of London*, October 14, 1854.

[47] Mary Agnes McCann, *The History of Mother Seton's Daughters: 1909-1917* (New York, NY: Longmans, Green & Co., 1917) p. 298.

[48] McCann, p. 300.

[49] McCann, p. 300.

[50] John Henry Lamott, *History of the Archdiocese of Cincinnati, 1821-1921*, (Cincinnati, OH: Frederick Pustet Company, Inc., 1921) p. 248.

[51] T. Sheppard, Jacob Deems and Peter Foy. *Report of the Commissioners of Health*, Baltimore City Health Department, 1815-1849. 1832. Maryland State Archives (Baltimore, MD).

[52] John J. Fialka, *Sisters: Catholic Nuns and the Making of America* (New York, NY: Macmillan, 2004) p. 61.

[53] Sister Mary Denis Maher, *To Bind the Wounds: Catholic Sister Nurses in the U.S. Civil War* (Baton Rouge, LA: LSU Press, 1999) pp. 38-39.

[54] Walter F. Atlee, "Review of Scrive's *Relation Medico-Chirugicale de la Campagne d'Orient*," *American Journal of the Medical Sciences* 42 (1861): 463-74.

[55] Freemon, p. 52.

[56] Mary Livermore, *What Shall We Tell Our Daughters: Superfluous Women and Other Lectures* (Boston, MA: Lee and Shepard, 1883) pp. 177-178.

CHAPTER 3

[1] Mary Massey, *Bonnet Brigades: American Woman and the Civil War* (New York: Knopf, 1966) p. 32.

[2] U.S. War Department, *The War of the Rebellion: A Compilation of the Official Records of the Union and Confederate Armies* (Washington, D.C.: U.S. Government Printing Office, 1880-1901), Series III, Part I, p. 107.

[3] George Worthington Adams, *Doctors in Blue, The Medical History of the Union Army in the Civil War* (New York, NY: Henry Schuman, 1952) p. 179.

[4] Agatha Young, *The Women and the Crisis: Women of the North in the Civil War* (New York, NY: McDowell, Oblesky, 1959) p. 99.

[5] Jane Stuart Woolsey, *Hospital Days, Reminiscence of a Civil War Nurse* (Roseville, MN: Edinborough Press, 1996) p. 4.

[6] Jeane Heimberger Candido, "Sisters and Nuns Who Were Nurses During the Civil War," *Blue and Gray Magazine*, October 1993.

[7] Francis Tiffany, *Life of Dorothea Lynde Dix* (New York, NY: Houghton Mifflin Company, 1918) p. 282-283.

[8] Tiffany, p. 282-283.

[9] Dorris Moore Lawson, *Dr. Mary E. Walker: A Biographical Sketch*, Master's Thesis, (Syracuse, NY: Syracuse University, 1954) p. 39.

[10] Agatha Young, *The Women and the Crisis: Women of the North in the Civil War* (New York, NY: McDowell, Obolensky, 1959) p. 98.

[11] John H. Brinton, *Personal Memoirs of John H. Brinton: Major and Surgeon, U.S.V.,* 1861-1865 (New York, NY: Neale Publishing Co., 1914) pp. 43-44.

[12] Brinton, p. 44.

[13] Brinton, pp. 44-45.

[14] Fialka, p. 62.

[15] Sarah Hopper Emerson, ed., *Abby Hopper Gibbons: Told Chiefly Through Her Correspondence, vol. II* (New York, NY: The Knickerbocker Press, 1896) p. 32.

[16] *Annals of the Civil War*, ASJPH, pp. 478-81. Note: This is a collection of first-person accounts of sisters' war-time experiences submitted by the Daughters of Charity following the war at the request of Father Francis Burlando.

[17] George Barton, *Angels of the Battlefield: A History of the Labors of the Catholic Sisterhoods in the Late Civil War* (Philadelphia, PA: The Catholic Art Publishing Company, 1897) pp. 29-30.

[18] Betty Ann McNeil, D.C., *Dear Masters: Extracts from Accounts by Sister Nurses* (Emmitsburg, MD: Seton Heritage Center, 2011) p. 77.

[19] McNeil, *Dear Masters*, p. 77.

CHAPTER 4

[1] *Mother Regina*, p. 92.

[2] *Mother Regina*, p. 92.

[3] *Mother Regina*, p. 93.

[4] *Mother Regina*, p. 72.

[5] *Mother Regina*, p. 73.

[6] *Mother Regina*, p. 75.

[7] *Mother Regina*, p. 76.

[8] *Mother Regina*, p. 84.

[9] *Mother Regina*, pp. 88-90.

CHAPTER 5

[1] *www.civilwarhome.com/ftsumter.htm* reprints the official record from *Confederate Military History*, Volume 5, Chapter 1.

[2] Brevet Major-General Samuel Crawford, *Genesis of the Civil War* (New York, NY: Charles L. Webster & Co., 1887) p. 443.

[3] Abraham Lincoln, Proclamation of Blockade Against Southern Ports, *www.historyplace.com/lincoln/proc-2.htm*

[4] ASJPH 3-3-5-1855:84.

[5] ASJPH 7-7-1-2.

[6] ASJPH 7-7-1-2.

[7] National Park Service: Petersburg National Battlefield VirtualCache Program, *www.nps.gov/pete/planyourvisit/upload/D2-Site-17-Mahone-Monument.pdf*

[8] Loyola Law and Betty Ann McNeil, *Daughters of Charity in the Civil War: Extracts from Personal Accounts of Sister Nurses* (2002 manuscript) p. 113. Note: This is a distilling of the Annals of the Civil War to focus on the first-person account of the Daughters of Charity that dealt directly with their war experiences.

[9] Law and McNeil, p. 113.

[10] Betty Ann McNeil, *Charity Afire Civil War Trilogy: Virginia* (Emmitsburg, MD: The National Shrine of Saint Elizabeth Ann Seton, 2011), p 26.

[11] Law and McNeil, p. 114.

[12] Law and McNeil, p. 114.

[13] Law and McNeil, p. 115.

[14] *Charleston Mercury*, July 24, 1861.

[15] McNeil, *Virginia*, p. 29.

[16] McNeil, *Virginia*, p. 29.

[17] John R. G. Hassard, *Life of the Most Reverend John Hughes, D.D., First Archbishop of New York with Extracts from his Private Correspondence* (New York, NY: D. Appleton & Co., 1866) p. 442.

[18] *Richmond Dispatch,* May 3, 1861.

[19] *Richmond Dispatch*, October 2, 1861.

[20] *Annals of the Civil War*, vol. II, ASJPH, p. 58. Note: This is a collection of first-person accounts of sisters' war-time experiences submitted by the Daughters of Charity following the war at the request of Father Francis Burlando.

[21] *Richmond Enquirer*, September 29, 1862.

[22] McNeil, *Dear Masters*, p. 153.

[23] Barton, p. 11.

[24] Barton, p. 11.

James Rada, Jr.

[25] McNeil, *Virginia*, p. 16.

[26] Barton, p. 12.

[27] Barton, pp. 12-13.

[28] Barton, p. 13.

[29] McNeil, p. 11.

[30] Barton, p. 13.

[31] Sister Matilda Coskery as quoted in *Enlightened Charity*, p. 372.

[32] Law and McNeil, p. 115.

[33] Barton, p. 16.

[34] McNeil, *Dear Masters*, p. 151.

[35] McNeil, *Dear Masters*, p. 151.

[36] Donald Dale Jackson and the Editors of Time-Life Books, *The Civil War: Twenty Million Yankees, The Northern Homefront* (Alexandria, VA: Time Life Books, 1985), p.8.

[37] Jackson, p.8.

[38] Harold Elk Staubing, *In Hospital and Camp: The Civil War Through the Eyes of Its Doctors and Nurses* (Mechanicsburg, PA: Stackpole Books, 1993) p. 95.

[39] Providence Hospital: History, *www.provhosp.org/About_Us/History.htm*

[40] Hannefin, pp. 70-71.

[41] Ellen Ryan Jolly, *Nuns of the Battlefield* (Providence, RI: The Providence Visitor Press, 1927) p. 60.

[42] *Washington Intelligencer*, June 5, 1861.

[43] Hannefin, pp. 117-118.

[44] Jolly, p. 70.

[45] Louisa May Alcott, *Hospital Sketches: An Army Nurse's True Account of her Experience during the Civil War* (Bedford, MA: Applewood Books) p. 27.

[46] Judith Harper, *Women During the Civil War: An Encyclopedia* (Boco Raton, FL: CRC Press, 2007) p. 75.

[47] Barton, pp. 43-4.

[48] Letter from Brig. General John Rathbone to Bishop McCloskey, June 1, 1861, ASJPH.

[49] *Annals, vol. II*, p. 52.

[50] *Blenkinsop*, p. 32.

[51] *Blenkinsop*, p. 33.

[52] *Annals, vol. II*, pp. 52-57.

[53] McNeil, *Virginia*, p. 19.

[54] Barton, p. 21.

[55] Sister Matilda Coskery as quoted in *Enlightened Charity*, p. 379.

[56] Barton, p. 21.

[57] Barton, p. 21.

[58] McNeil, *Virginia*, p. 20.
[59] McNeil, *Virginia*, p. 20.
[60] *Annals, vol. II*, p. 52.
[61] Edmund J. Raus, Jr., *Ministering Angel: The Reminiscences of Harriet A. Dada, a Union Army Nurse in the Civil War* (Gettysburg, PA: Thomas Publications, 2004) p. 18.
[62] Barton, p. 23.
[63] *Annals, vol. II*, p. 52-57.
[64] Barton, p. 24.
[65] *Blenkinsop*, p. 33.

CHAPTER 6

[1] George W. Adams, *Doctors in Blue: The Medical History of the Union Army in the Civil War* (New York, NY: Henry Schuman, 1952) p. 129.
[2] Sister Matilda Coskery as quoted in *Enlightened Charity*, p. 379.
[3] Hannefin, p. 70.
[4] Frank R. Freemon, *Gangrene and Glory: Medical Care During the American Civil War* (Urbana, IL: University of Illinois Press, 2001) p. 46.
[5] Hannefin, p. 114.
[6] Freemon, p. 36.
[7] Providence Hospital History, *www.provhosp.org/About_us/History.htm*
[8] Freemon, p. 30.
[9] Sarah Hopper Emerson, ed., *Abby Hopper Gibbons: Told Chiefly Through Her Correspondence, vol. I* (New York, NY: The Knickerbocker Press, 1897) p. 324.
[10] Edward O. Hewitt, "A Letter from a British Military Observer of the American Civil War," *Military Affairs 16,* 1952.
[11] *Annals, vol. II,* pp. 58-59.
[12] Hannefin, p. 135.
[13] Barton, p. 14.
[14] Barton, p. 14.
[15] Barton, pp. 14-15.
[16] Barton, p. 15.
[17] *Charleston Mercury,* July 24, 1861.
[18] *Charleston Mercury,* August 14, 1861.
[19] *Annals, vol. II,* p. 111.
[20] Missouri Civil War Museum: A Few Fascinating Missouri Civil War Facts, *www.mcwm.org/history_facts.html*
[21] Barton, p. 28.
[22] Barton, p. 28.

James Rada, Jr.

[23] *Notes of the Sisters' Services in Military Hospitals, 1861-1865*, ASJPH, Emmitsburg, MD, p. 49.

[24] *Annals, vol. II*, p. 128.

[25] Civil War in Missouri Facts, *home.usmo.com/~momollus/MOFACTS.HTM*

[26] Barton, pp. 29-30.

[27] Barton, pp. 32, 33.

[28] Law and McNeil, p. 50.

[29] Barton, pp. 33-34.

[30] *Blenkinsop,* p. 35.

[31] *Charleston Mercury,* August 20, 1861.

[32] *Annals, vol. II*, p. 62.

[33] *Charleston Mercury*, September 21, 1861.

[34] *Annals, vol. I*, pp. 506-518.

[35] Letter from Father Burlando to the Daughters of Charity, undated, ASJPH 7-1-7:9.

[36] Letter from Burlando to Daughters of Charity, undated.

[37] Letter from Burlando to Daughters of Charity, undated.

[38] *Mother Regina*, p. 60.

CHAPTER 7

[1] Ellin M. Kelly, *Numerous Choirs: A Chronicle of Elizabeth Bayley Seton and Her Spiritual Daughters, Volume II: Expansion, Division, and War 1861-1865*, (Saint Meinrad, IN: Abbey Press, 1996) p. 216.

[2] U.S. Library of Congress, *www.loc.gov/teachers/classroommaterials/presentationsandactivities/presenta tions/immigration/irish2.html*

[3] Catholic Encyclopedia, *www.catholicity.com/b/blenkinsop.html*

[4] *Blenkinsop*, pp. 6-7.

[5] *Blenkinsop*, p. 5.

[6] *Blenkinsop*, p. 9.

[7] *Blenkinsop*, p. 11.

[8] *Blenkinsop*, p. 13.

[9] *Blenkinsop*, p. 13.

[10] *Blenkinsop*, p. 15.

[11] *Blenkinsop*, p. 19.

[12] *Blenkinsop*, p. 21.

[13] *Blenkinsop*, pp. 23-24.

[14] *Blenkinsop*, pp. 28-29.

[15] *Blenkinsop*, p. 30.

[16] ASJPH 3-3-5-1861:278.

[17] *Blenkinsop, p. 35.*

[18] *Blenkinsop, p. 36.*

[19] *Blenkinsop, p. 36*

[20] *Blenkinsop, p. 37-39.*

[21] *Blenkinsop, p. 37-39.*

[22] *Blenkinsop, p. 37-39.*

[23] A visitor is a regional superior priest who visits the priest of the mission for administrative and pastoral reasons.

[24] *Blenkinsop, p. 39-40.*

[25] *Blenkinsop, p. 40.*

[26] *Annals, vol. II,* p. 478.

CHAPTER 8

[1] Letter from Sister Francis McGinnis to Father Burlando, January 8, 1862, Archives of Seton Provincialate (ASP), Los Altos Hills, CA, *Correspondence of the Director.*

[2] Letter from McGinnis to Burlando, January 8, 1862.

[3] McNeil, *Virginia*, p. 30; *Annals, vol. II,* p. 66.

[4] *Blenkinsop*, p. 40.

[5] Barton, p. 71.

[6] *Blenkinsop,* p. 40.

[7] Kelly, p. 223.

[8] National Park Service: Exchange Hotel, *nps.gov/history/nr/travel/journey/exc.htm*

[9] *Annals, vol. II,* p. 66.

[10] *Blenkinsop,* pp. 41-42.

[11] *Blenkinsop,* pp. 41-42.

[12] *Blenkinsop,* p. 42.

[13] *Annals, vol. II,* pp. 67-68.

[14] *Mother Regina,* pp. 108-109.

[15] ASJPH 7-10-14:55.

[16] ASJPH 7-10-14:56.

[17] Sara Trainer Smith, ed., "Notes on Satterlee Military Hospital, West Philadelphi, Penna. from 1862 Until Its Close in 1865 from the Journal Kept at the Hospital by a Sister of Charity," *Records of the American Catholic Historical Society of Philadelphia, Volume 8* (1897): 400.

[18] *Notes on Sisters' Services,* p. 394.

[19] Barton, p. 106.

[20] *Notes on Sisters' Services,* p. 394.

[21] Smith, p. 400.

[22] *Notes on Sisters' Services,* p. 394.

[23] *Notes on Sisters' Services,* p. 394.

[24] Smith, pp. 401-2.

[25] Smith, p. 405.

[26] *Notes on Sisters' Services,* p. 401.

[27] *Notes on Sisters' Services,* p. 401.

[28] Hannefin, p. 115. This site would eventually become Arlington National Cemetery when the Federal Government started burying dead there in 1864 after it acquired the land without due process.

[29] Jolly, pp. 60-61.

[30] Jane Turn Censer, ed., *The Papers of Frederick Law Olmsted, Vol. 4, Defending the Union* (Baltimore: Johns Hopkins University Press, 1986) pp. 30-31.

[31] Jeane Heimberger Candido, "Sisters and Nuns Who Were Nurses During the Civil War" *Blue and Gray,* Oct. 1993.

[32] Letter from Father Francis Burlando to Mother Ann Simeon, June 23, 1862 as quoted in *Mother Regina,* p. 102.

[33] Letter from Father Francis Burlando to Mother Ann Simeon, June 23, 1862 as quoted in *Mother Regina,* p. 103.

[34] Letter from Father Francis Burlando to Mother Ann Simeon, June 23, 1862 as quoted in *Mother Regina,* p. 103.

[35] *Annals, vol. I,* p. 19.

[36] Hannefin, p. 115.

[37] *Annals, vol. I,* pp. 19-20.

[38] Letter from Father Francis Burlando to Mother Ann Simeon, June 23, 1862 as quoted in *Mother Regina,* p. 103.

[39] *Mother Regina,* pp. 103-104.

[40] *Notes on Sisters' Services,* pp. 63-64.

[41] Letter from Spencer Glasgow Welch to his wife, June 29, 1862, as quoted in *In Hospital and Camp: The Civil War through the eyes of its doctors and nurses,* Harold Elk Straubing (Mechanicsburg, PA: Stackpole Books, 1993) p. 64.

[42] Law and McNeil, p. 121.

CHAPTER 9

[1] Betty Ann McNeil, *Charity Afire Civil War Trilogy: Maryland* (Emmitsburg, MD: The National Shrine of Saint Elizabeth Ann Seton, 2011), p. 13.

[2] Barton, p. 56.

[3] Libster and McNeil, p. 378.

[4] McNeil, *Maryland,* p. 15.

[5] Barton, p. 56.

[6] *Annals, vol. I*, pp. 29-30.

[7] Libster and McNeil, p. 378.

[8] Libster and McNeil, p. 398.

[9] Louise Sullivan, DC, ed. and trans., *Louise de Marillac Spiritual Writings: Correspondence and Thoughts* (New York: New York City Press, 1991) p. 763.

[10] William Stokes, *38th Annual Report of the Mount Hope Retreat*, ASJPH, Emmitsburg, MD, p. 19.

[11] Amariah Brigham, "Editorial Correspondence," *American Journal of Insanity 5, no. 1* (1848), Archives of the American Psychiatric Association.

[12] Sister Betty Ann McNeil and Martha Libster wrote about the difficulties of trying to date the manuscript in *Enlightened Charity.* They considered handwriting and textual references, but the best that they can come up with Is that it was most likely written prior to 1850, though some of the evidences disputes even this.

CHAPTER 10

[1] Point Lookout State Park History, *www.dnr.state.md.us/publiclands/ptlookouthistory.asp*

[2] Point Lookout State Park: Hammond General Hospital, *www.hmdb.org/marker.asp?marker=1001*

[3] Point Lookout State Park: Hammond General Hospital, *www.hmdb.org/marker.asp?marker=1001*

[4] Point Lookout Prisoner of War Camp, *www.americanwars101.com/pow/md-point-lookout.html*

[5] *Annals, vol. I*, p. 23.

[6] McNeil, *Dear Masters*, p. 45.

[7] *Mother Regina*, p. 105.

[8] Letter from Sister Regina Smith to Mother Gilberte-Elise Montcellet, August 11, 1862, as quoted in *Remarks on Our Deceased Sisters (*1863), 27-28. *Remarks on Our Deceased Sisters* was an annual publication that was translated and printed at the Central House in Emmitsburg, MD, from 1852 to 1867.

[9] Hannefin, p. 132.

[10] McNeil, *Dear Masters*, p. 57.

[11] *Annals, vol. I,* pp. 1-2.

[12] McNeil, *Dear Masters*, p. 57.

[13] Law and McNeil, p. 37.

[14] Smith, p. 401.

[15] McNeil, *Dear Masters*, p. 55.

James Rada, Jr.

[16] McNeil, *Dear Masters*, p. 55.
[17] McNeil, *Dear Masters*, pp. 55-56.
[18] McNeil, *Dear Masters*, p. 56.
[19] *Annals, vol.* II, p. 98.

CHAPTER 11

[1] Robert E. Lee as quoted in *The Bloodiest Day: The Battle of Antietam,* William C. Davis and the Editors of Time-Life Books (Alexandria, VA: Time-Life Books, 1983) p. 89.
[2] Jacob Engelbrecht, The Diary of Jacob Engelbrecht, William R. Quyunn, ed., September 5, 1862 (Frederick, MD: The Historical Society of Frederick County, 1976).
[3] *The (Frederick) Examiner*, September 24, 1862.
[4] Thomas John Chew Williams and Folger McKinsey, *History of Frederick County, Maryland* (Baltimore: Regional Publishing Company, 1979) p. 376.
[5] Barton, p. 59.; McNeil, *Maryland*, p. 18.
[6] Catherine Thomas Markell, *Diary*, September 8, 1862, C. Burr Artz Public Library, Frederick, MD.
[7] Lewis H. Steiner, M.D., *Report of Lewis H. Steiner, M.D.* (New York, NY: Anson D.F. Randolph, 1862) p. 8.
[8] Alexander Hunter, "A High Private's Account of the Battle of Sharpsburg," *Southern Historical Society Papers, vol. X*, p. 508.
[9] Barton, p. 60.
[10] Barton, pp. 60-61.
[11] Katherine E. Coon, *The Sisters of Charity in Nineteenth-Century America: Civil War Nurses and Philanthropic Pioneers,* Thesis for the Departments of History and Philanthropic Studies, Indiana University, May 2010, pp. 110-1.
[12] Barton, pp. 60-61.
[13] McNeil, *Maryland,* p. 19.
[14] *Annals, vol. I*, p. 34.
[15] McNeil, *Maryland,* p. 20.
[16] *Annals, vol. II*, p. 69.
[17] Law and McNeil, p. 13.
[18] Barton, p. 74.
[19] Law and McNeil, p. 13.
[20] Law and McNeil, p. 13.
[21] Libster and McNeil, p. 379.
[22] Law and McNeil, p. 16.
[23] Law and McNeil, p. 16.
[24] Barton, p. 78.

[25] Barton, p. 76.
[26] Barton, p. 75.
[27] Law and McNeil, p. 14.
[28] McNeil, *Dear Masters*, p. 20.
[29] Barton, p. 76.
[30] McNeil, *Maryland*, p. 21.
[31] Letter from Francis Burlando to Mother Gilberte-Elise Montcellet, September 1, 1862, as quoted in *Remarks on Our Deceased Sisters*, (1863) 29.
[32] Surgical Reminiscences of the Civil War by W.W. Keen, M.D. Professor of Surgery, Jefferson Medical, *www.civilwarsurgeons.org/articles/written_by_participants/surgical_reminiscences.pdf*
[33] Letter from Father Francis Burlando to Sister Elizabeth Montcellet as quoted in *Numerous Choirs: A Chronicle of Elizabeth Bayley Seton and Her Spiritual Daughters, Volume II: Expansion, Division, and War 1861-1865*, (Saint Meinrad, IN: Abbey Press, 1996) p. 226.
[34] *Richmond Enquirer*, June 11, 1862.
[35] Law and McNeil, p. 108.
[36] Smith, p. 410.
[37] *Galveston Weekly News*, October 29, 1862.
[38] Fialka, p. 63.
[39] *Provincial Annals (1846-1871)*, ASJPH, pp. 540-541.

CHAPTER 12

[1] *Annals, vol. II*, p. 106.
[2] McNeil, *Dear Masters*, p. 13.
[3] McNeil, *Dear Masters*, p. 13.
[4] 3-3-5-1863, ASJPH, p. 302.
[5] Barton, p. 87.
[6] Barton, pp. 87-88.
[7] Barton, p. 88.
[8] Law and McNeil, p. 2.
[9] *Annals*, pp. 48-49.
[10] Law and McNeil, p. 3.
[11] Law and McNeil, p. 3.
[12] Barton, pp. 90-91.
[13] *Mother Regina*, p. 114.
[14] James Helman, *History of Emmitsburg, Maryland* (1906) reprinted by the Emmitsburg Area Historical Society,

James Rada, Jr.

www.emmitsburg.net/archive_list/articles/history/helmans/helmans_81-90.htm#Fires
[15] Michael Hillman, "The Great Fire of 1863," Emmitsburg Area Historical Society, *www.emmitsburg.net/archive_list/articles/history/stories/great_fire_of_1863.htm*
[16] Helman, *History of Emmitsburg, Maryland.*
[17] Hillman, "The Great Fire of 1863."
[18] Robert M. Preston, "The Great Fire of Emmitsburg," Emmitsburg Area Historical Society, *www.emmitsburg.net/archive_list/articles/history/stories/emmitsburg_fire.htm*
[19] Sister John Mary Crumlish, *1809-1959*, ASJPH (1959), p. 94.
[20] Preston, "The Great Fire of Emmitsburg."
[21] *Annals of St. Joseph's*, ASJPH, pp. 520-521.
[22] Regis de Trobriand, *Four Years with the Army of the Potomac*, trans. George W. Dauchy (Boston, MA: Ticknor and Company, 1889) pp. 485-487.
[23] de Trobiand, pp. 485-487.
[24] *Annals of St. Joseph's*, p. 532.
[25] *Annals of St. Joseph's*, p. 529.
[26] Law and McNeil, p. 20.
[27] *Annals of St. Joseph's*, p. 533.
[28] *Annals,* pp. 527-528.
[29] *Annals*, pp. 524.
[30] *Annals*, pp. 534.
[31] McEntee, pp. 45-46.
[32] Despite the fact that the Daughters of Charity records list June 30 as the date for this, it seems unlikely. No other corroborating evidence has been found. Though the incident happened, it is more likely that it occurred in 1864 when General J.E.B. Stuart was seen in town with his men.
[33] *Annals of St. Joseph's*, p. 561.
[34] *Annals of St. Joseph's*, pp. 524-525.
[35] Letter from Emma M. to May Preston, August 23, 1863, MS 978 Manuscripts collection, Maryland Historical Society.
[36] *Annals of St. Joseph's*, p. 525.
[37] Barton, p. 93.
[38] Letter from Father Francis Burlando to Father Jean Baptiste Etienne, Superior General of the Vincentians, July 8, 1863, as quoted in *Mother Regina and Mother Ann Simeon*, p. 116.

CHAPTER 13

[1] Letter from Father Francis Burlando to Father Jean Baptiste Etienne, Superior General of the Vincentians, July 8, 1863.

[2] Kelly, pp. 228-229.

[3] CWSAC Battle Summaries: Gettysburg, *www.nps.gov/history/hps/abpp/battles/pa002.htm*

[4] *Mother Regina*, p. 129.

[5] Sister Eleanor Casey, "The Daughters of Charity of Emmitsburg & the Battle of Gettysburg," Greater Emmitsburg Area Historical Society, *www.emmitsburg.net/archive_list/articles/history/civil_war/doc_civil_war.htm*

[6] *Mother Regina*, p. 130.

[7] *Annals*, pp. 535, 561.

[8] Father Burlando as quoted in *Numerous Choirs*, p. 235.

[9] *Annals, vol. I,* p. 536.

[10] *Annals, vol. I,* p. 562.

[11] *Mother Regina, p. 131.*

[12] *Provincial Annals,* pp. 537-538.

[13] *Mother Regina*, p. 131.

[14] *Annals, vol. I,* pp. 562-563.

[15] Jonathan Letterman, "Report on the Operations of the Medical Department during the Battle of Gettysburg." *MSH, Medical Volume, pt. 1*, appendix, pp.140-2.

[16] *Mother Regina*, p. 132; Betty Ann McNeil, *Charity Afire Civil War Trilogy: Pennsylvania* (Emmitsburg, MD: The National Shrine of Saint Elizabeth Ann Seton, 2011), p 3.

[17] *Annals, vol. I,* pp. 539-540.

[18] Sister M. Liguori, H.F.N. "Polish Sisters in the Civil War," *Polish American Studies* 7:1-2 (1950) ASJPH 7-5-1-1, #17.

[19] *Mother Regina*, p. 133.

[20] *Mother Regina*, pp. 133-134.

[21] *Mother Regina*, p. 134.

[22] *Mother Regina*, p. 134.

[23] Law and McNeil, p. 71.

[24] *Mother Regina*, p. 135; McNeil, *Pennsylvania*, p. 4.

[25] *Mother Regina*, p. 135.

[26] *Mother Regina*, p. 135.

[27] *Mother Regina*, p. 136-137.

[28] *Mother Regina*, p. 137.

[29] *Mother Regina*, pp. 137-138.

James Rada, Jr.

[30] *Mother Regina*, p. 138.
[31] Pennsylvania College became Gettysburg College in 1921.
[32] Barton, p. 98.
[33] *Mother Regina*, p. 139.
[34] *Mother Regina*, pp. 139-140.
[35] *Mother Regina*, p. 140.
[36] *Mother Regina*, pp. 140-141.
[37] *Mother Regina*, p. 141-142.
[38] *Satterlee notebook*, manuscript. ASJPH, pp. 50-51.
[39] Smith, pp. 408-409.
[40] Sister Marie De Lourdes Walsh, *The Sisters of Charity of New York: 1809-1959, vol. 1* (New York, NY: Fordham University Press, 1960) p. 201.
[41] *Blenkinsop*, pp. 44-45.
[42] *Blenkinsop*, p. 45.
[43] *Blenkinsop*, pp. 44-45.
[44] *Blenkinsop*, pp. 44-45.
[45] William G. Stevenson as quoted in *In Hospital and Camp*, p. 29.
[46] William G. Stevenson as quoted in *In Hospital and Camp*, p. 30.
[47] William G. Stevenson as quoted in *In Hospital and Camp*, p. 31.
[48] William G. Stevenson as quoted in *In Hospital and Camp*, p. 31.
[49] Point Lookout State Park: Hammond General Hospital.
[50] Point Lookout State Park History.
[51] Point Lookout State Park History.
[52] Congregational Archives of the Sisters of the Holy Cross, Saint Mary's, Notre Dame, IN (ACSC), Copy of General Order 351, Oct. 29, 1863.
[53] *Annals, vol. I*, p. 23.
[54] Gibbons, *Hopper, vol. 1*, pp. 347-8.
[55] McNeil, *Maryland*, p. 30.
[56] ASJPH 333-5-1863, p. 326.

CHAPTER 14

[1] *Mother Regina*, p. 61.
[2] *Mother Regina*, pp. 62-3.
[3] *Mother Regina*, p. 63.
[4] Hannefin, p. 135.
[5] *Mother Regina*, p. 66.
[6] ASJPH 3-3-5-1864, pp. 329-30.
[7] *Provincial Annals*, pp. 565-566.
[8] *Mother Regina*, p. 156.
[9] McNeil, *Dear Masters*, p. 7.

[10] McNeil, *Dear Masters*, p. 7.
[11] Civil War Prisons: Alton Prison (Union), *www.factasy.com/civil_war/book/export/html/459*
[12] McNeil, *Dear Masters*, p. 7.
[13] Civil War Prisons: Alton Prison (Union).
[14] Law and McNeil, p. 5.
[15] McNeil, *Dear Masters*, p. 8.
[16] ASJPH 3-3-5-1864, p. 332; *Annals, vol. I*, pp. 4-5.
[17] *Provincial Annals*, p. 570.
[18] *Annals, vol. I*, pp. 5-6.
[19] Law and McNeil, p. 7.
[20] *Mother Regina*, pp. 158-159.
[21] Daniel Shipman Troy, "How I Became a Catholic," ASJPH 10-1-20.
[22] Smith, p. 413.
[23] Smith, p. 410.
[24] Barton, pp. 110-111.
[25] Barton, pp. 111-112.
[26] U.S. War Department, *The Wars of the Rebellion: A Compilation of the Official Records of the Union and Confederate Armies, part 2, vol. 7* (Washington, DC: Government Printing Office, 1880-1901) pp. 221, 373.
[27] National Park Service: The Battle of Monocacy: Aftermath, *www.nps.gov/mono/historyculture/battle_aftermath.htm*
[28] McNeil, *Dear Masters*, p. 42.
[29] Edward McPherson, *A political history of the united states during the great rebellion* (Washington, DC: Philp & Solomons, 1865) p. 541.
[30] Wm. H. Elder, *Character-glimpses of Most Reverend William Henry Elder: Second Archbishop of Cincinnati* (Cincinnati, OH: Frederick Pustet & Company, 1911) pp. 53-4.
[31] Crumlish, p. 94.
[32] *Annals, vol. I*, pp. 24-25; McNeil, *Maryland*, p. 31.
[33] McNeil, *Maryland*, p. 31.
[34] *Annals, vol. I*, pp. 24-25; McNeil, *Maryland*, p. 31.
[35] McNeil, *Maryland*, p. 32.
[36] McNeil, *Dear Masters*, pp. 50-51.
[37] McNeil, *Dear Masters*, p. 52.
[38] McNeil, *Dear Masters*, p. 52.
[39] McNeil, *Dear Masters*, p. 52.
[40] McNeil, *Dear Masters*, p. 53.
[41] McNeil, *Dear Masters*, p. 53.
[42] *Provincial Annals*, p. 572.
[43] *Annals, vol. I*, p. 39.

James Rada, Jr.

44 Smith, p. 426.
45 ASJPH 3-3-5-1864, p. 353.

CHAPTER 15

1 *Annals, vol. I*, pp. 478-481.
2 Smith, p. 428.
3 Law and McNeil, p. 84.
4 *Annals, vol. II*, p. 68.
5 *Richmond Dispatch*, June 3, 1864.
6 *Provincial Annals*, p. 581.
7 "Washington and Georgetown, D.C.," *Indexes to Field Records of Hospitals, 1821-1912*, Manuscript Record Group 94, National Archives.
8 *Annals, vol. I*, pp. 11-13.
9 ASJPH 3-3-5-1865, pp. 358-359.
10 *Provincial Annals*, p. 581.
11 Abraham Lincoln Second Inaugural Address, *www.bartleby.com/124/pres32.html*
12 *Notes on Sisters' Serivces*, pp. 64-65.
13 The Price in Blood! Casualties in the Civil War, *www.civilwarhome.com/casualties.htm*
14 ASJPH 3-3-5-1865, pp. 368-370.
15 Smith, p. 408.
16 *Annals, vol. I*, p. 27.
17 McNeil, *Maryland*, p. 34.
18 ASJPH 3-3-5-1865, p. 372.
19 ASJPH 3-3-5-1865, p. 372.

CHAPTER 16

1 Father Burlando as quoted in *Mother Euphemia Blenkinsop*, pp. 47-54.
2 *Sandusky Star-Journal*, September 29, 1924.
3 *Sandusky Star-Journal*, September 29, 1924.

APPENDICES

1 Original notes provided by the Daughters of Charity, Emmitsburg, MD.
2 American Civil War Battle Statistics: Commanders and Casualties, *americancivilwar.com/cwstats.html*
3 Maher, pp. 69-70; McNeil, *Maryland*, p. *v*; Jolly, pp. 1, 19, 36, 57, 85, 93, 101, 111, 124, 158, 170, 181, 206, 223, 240, 258, 271, 287, 299, 309, 320.

Made in the USA
Middletown, DE
11 November 2023

42354979R00130